Chair Yoga

FOR SENIORS

Over 60

10-Minute *Daily Routine with*

STEP-BY-STEP INSTRUCTIONS

IMPROVE BALANCE, FLEXIBILITY AND MINDFULNESS

JONATHAN PRICE

JONATHAN PRICE

is an independent publisher, if you enjoy this book, please consider supporting us by leaving a review!

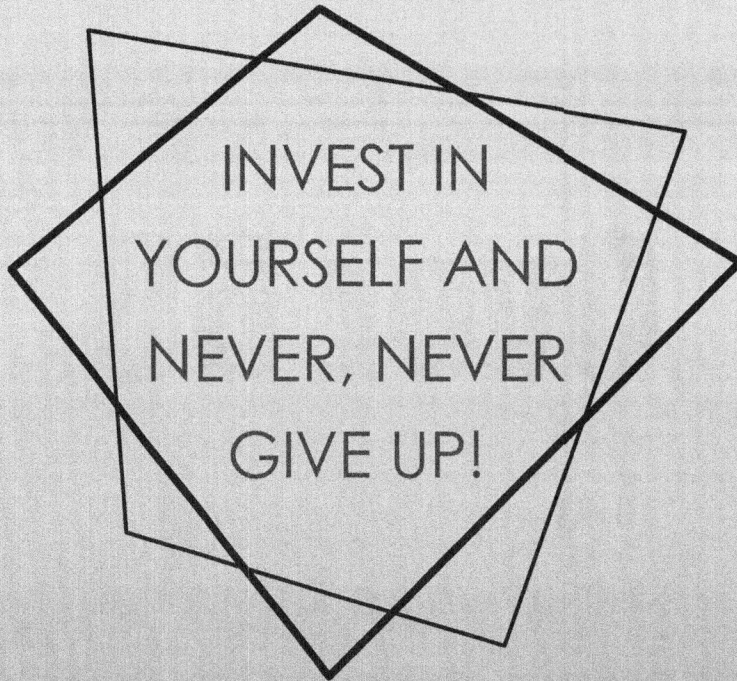

INVEST IN YOURSELF AND NEVER, NEVER GIVE UP!

THANK YOU FOR PURCHASING THIS BOOK,

IF YOU ENJOY THIS TITLE,

THEN FEEDBACK ON AMAZON WOULD BE

GREATLY APPRECIATED.

If you are not satisfied with this book, then drop us an email at:
selfcareemotional@gmail.com

We want our books to be truly enjoyable for everyone.

Table of Contents

INTRODUCTION 8

HOW TO USE THIS BOOK 11

CHAPTER ONE: BREATHING TECHNIQUES (PRANAYAMA) 15

    ALTERNATE NOSTRIL BREATHING (NADI SHODHANA) 16

    OCEAN BREATH (UJJAYI PRANAYAMA) 17

    CLEANSING BREATH (KAPALBHATI) 18

    BELLOWS BREATH (BHASTRIKA) 19

    BREATH RETENTION (KUMBHAKA) 20

    COOLING BREATH (SITALI) 21

    HISSING TEETH BREATH (SITKARI) 22

CHAPTER TWO: WARM-UP EXERCISES 23

    CHAIR MOUNTAIN POSE (CHAIR TADASANA) 24

    SEATED NECK ROLLS (KANTASANCHALANA) 25

    CHAIR CAT-COW STRETCH (CHAIR MARJARYASANA BITILASANA) ... 27

    PELVIC TILTS/CIRCLES 28

    FOOT AND ANKLE STRETCH 29

    SEATED SHOULDER ROLLS 30

    SEATED SIDE BEND POSE 31

    SUN SALUTATIONS 32

    MARCHING FLOW 33

    KNEE SWINGS 34

CHAPTER THREE: OUR SPECIALIZED INTRODUCTORY PROGRAM FOR ABSOLUTE BEGINNERS .35

    BREATHING EXERCISE 36

    WARM UP YOUR BODY 37

    UPPER BODY EXERCISES 38

    ASSISTED NECK STRETCH 39

    UP-DOWN, RIGHT-LEFT (EYE MOVEMENT) 40

    WIDE SMILES 41

    SHOULDER SHRUGS 42

Elbow Extensions 43

Arm Circles 44

Hand pulls.. 45

Wrist Extensions 46

Torso and Lower Body Exercises.. 47

Seated Forward Bend 48

Single Leg Stretch... 49

Warrior I (Virabhadrasana I).. 51

Chair Downward Facing Dog (Adho Mukha Svanasana) 53

Leg lifts... 54

Seated Knee Hugs 55

Seated Heel Raises.. 56

Toe raises 57

Standing Chair Warrior I.. 58

Cooling Down 59

Cooling Breath (Sithali).. 60

Final Relaxation and Meditation 61

CHAPTER FOUR: OUR DEDICATED INTERMEDIATE PROGRAM 63

Cleansing Breath (Kapalbhati)... 64

Seated Head Tilt 65

Close/Open (Eye Movement).. 66

Open wide (Mouth movement) 67

Shoulder Rotations 68

High Altar Arms... 69

Finger Extensions 70

Wrist Rotations.. 71

Eagle Arms (Chair Garudasana) 72

Extended Side Angle 73

Standing Forward Fold 74

Seated Twist 75

Chair Pigeon Pose 76

Knee to Chest Pose (Eka Pada Apanasana).. 77

Chair Goddess Pose (Chair Utkata Konasana) 78

Cross-Legged Side Bend 79

Warrior II (Virabhadrasana II) 80

Quad Stretch 82

Feet Point and Flex 83

Calf Stretch.. 84

Cooling Down 85

Cooling Breath (Sithali).. 86

Final Relaxation and Meditation 87

CHAPTER FIVE: OUR EXCLUSIVE ADVANCED PROGRAM 89

Breathing Exercise... 90

Seated Head Circles.. 91

EYE CIRCLES...92

SIDES-TO-SIDES WITH LOWER JAW (MOUTH MOVEMENT) 93

SHOULDER SWINGS..94

HIGH ALTAR SIDE LEANS 95

UPSIDE-DOWNSIDE FINGER EXTENSIONS..96

SEAT LIFTS...97

INTENSE SIDE STRETCH (PARSVOTTANASANA) 98

CHAIR BOAT POSE (CHAIR NAVASANA) 99

CHAIR GODDESS TWIST (CHAIR PARIVRTTA UTKATA KONASANA) 100

WARRIOR III (VIRABHADRASANA III)...101

CROSS-LEGGED TWIST..102

ADVANCED HAMSTRING STRETCH...103

HIGH LUNGE 104

TREE...105

RAISED KNEE BALANCE..106

TIPPY TOES..107

COOLING DOWN..109

COOLING BREATH (SITKARI)...111

LAXATION AND MEDITATION 113

CHAPTER SIX: BEGINNER PROGRAM FOR OSTEOARTHRITIS OF THE HANDS, KNEES, AND HIPS
....**115**

BREATHING EXERCISE...116

HAND PULLS...117

FINGER EXTENSIONS..119

WRIST EXTENSIONS 121

ELBOW EXTENSIONS..123

SHOULDER SHRUGS...124

HANDS ON SHOULDER ROLLS..126

SEATED FORWARD BEND 128

KNEE SWINGS...130

SINGLE LEG ANKLE CIRCLES..132

COOLING POSE: LEGS ON A CHAIR (SAVASANA VARIATION) 134

FINAL RELAXATION AND MEDITATION..136

CHAPTER SEVEN: INTERMEDIATE PROGRAM FOR OSTEOARTHRITIS OF THE HANDS, KNEES, AND HIPS...**139**

BREATHING EXERCISE...140

ALTERNATING ARM RAISES WITH WEIGHTS 142

SHOULDER ROTATIONS...144

HIGH ALTAR ARMS 145

WRIST ROTATIONS...146

SEATED KNEE HUGS...147

RAISED KNEE BALANCE..148

OPPOSITE LEG AND KNEE LIFT (VYAGHRASANA VARIATION) 150

SIT TO STAND...152

SEATED TWIST 154

FINAL RELAXATION POSE 156

CONCLUSION **158**

REFERENCES **159**

Introduction

Staying active is key to good health and well-being. It is even more important for seniors because it helps in impeding age-related challenges. While performing the normal workouts or exercises like strength training to stay active can be perfect for your health, it can be a little harder for seniors. The risks of falls, injuries, joint pain, or strains are higher among older people. Besides, it is difficult for the elderly to get the incentive to want to go for a long run or gym. Here is where yoga steps in.

Seniors can stay active and improve muscle strength and flexibility while lowering the risks of falls, muscle strains, and other injuries by performing yoga exercises. Yoga has been proven in several studies to have numerous benefits for the elderly. Not just the elderly, but yoga is truly beneficial to anyone. If you are already strong and healthy, practicing yoga will help you maintain your muscle strength and health status. And if you have some health problems, whether old age-related or not, temporary or chronic, practicing yoga will help you regain good health and the strength and stability that has been compromised by your condition.

Yoga can be done by anyone. However, due to the different levels of difficulty and an intricate repertoire of ancient yoga, practicing traditional yoga can be daunting to people who are not steady on their feet, those who are new to the idea, those who want to start slowly, or those who would just feel more confident sitting down. This is especially true for seniors and those with mobility problems. The good news is that yoga has exercises for every skill group, and if you fall into this group of people, chair yoga is the best for you.

Chair yoga is a type of Hatha branch of yoga. Hatha is the yoga of the body that includes poses, breathing, and meditation. Chair yoga can be done either sitting for the entire session or in some classes standing and using the chair as a prop for balance. One of the greatest things about Chair yoga is that it can be practiced by people of any size, age, shape, ability, level of activity, those with past injuries, chronic conditions, weight problems, disabilities, or anyone who wants to increase his or her range of motion through gradual and gentle exercises. In other words, anyone can practice chair yoga. Seniors can enjoy all the benefits of yoga without having to get up and down off of the floor or stressing their joints through the practice of yoga using chairs.

Chair yoga cultivates a mind-body connection, helping you create a better harmony between your body, mind, and spirit. Besides, seniors who practice chair yoga enjoy improved flexibility and stability that comes with it. Flexibility and balance are very important in performing most of the daily tasks and movements. Most seniors experience occasional or sometimes chronic foot pain or numbness. Not forgetting the obvious joint pain. Since feet and joints are the foundation of your mobility, most seniors experience limited mobility, which is the major culprit of increased risk of falls among the elderly. A properly done chair yoga emphasizes feet and joints, stretching and strengthening them. Holding a pose for several breaths also helps relax and loosen your muscles and connective tissues which helps increase your range of motion. A study published in the international journal of therapy shows that practicing chair yoga can dramatically boost the overall flexibility of older adults (Ferinatti, et al. 2014).

Another important benefit of chair yoga in seniors is increased bone and body strength. So, if you are worried about brittle bones and osteoarthritis, get hooked on yoga classes. A consistent yoga routine can help boost bone strength and strengthen your entire body. Promising research conducted among postmenopausal women suggested that performing yoga can improve bone density (Harvard Health, 2022). Seniors with strong bones are flexible and less prone to falls.

Reduced stress and anxiety, and enhanced breathing are also common among people who practice yoga, including the elderly who practice chair yoga. All types of yoga inherently require you to be mindful of your breathing and ensure meditative movements. By doing so, you shift your focus from stressful thoughts to the present thus creating a sense of peace and promoting relaxation. Research conducted on cortisol and antidepressant effects of yoga demonstrated that yoga helps lower the levels of the stress hormone cortisol and also reduces anxiety symptoms (Thirthalli et al. 2013).

A survey conducted by the National Institute of Health Survey also indicates that 85% of people who reported having been practicing yoga said they experienced reduced stress as a result (Wellness-related…2012). The breathing control practice of yoga helps expand the capacity of your lungs thus improving your pulmonary health. A study conducted on yoga's influence on the pulmonary function of elderly women found that those women who practiced yoga three times each week for 12 weeks experienced significant improvement in their heart function (Bezera et al. 2014).

Yoga also helps boost confidence and reduces depression. Most seniors are left alone with no family to live with. This experience can result in loneliness and stress and then turn into depression. Yoga can help decrease the symptoms of depression among all ages including seniors who are over 60 (Bridges & Sharma, 2017).

Most seniors complain of sleep disturbances. Yoga can help you with this. If you have trouble sleeping during the night, try yoga. Just like any other exercise or type of yoga, chair yoga can help regulate the circadian rhythm of your body and improve sleep quality. It provides just the right amount of exertion without getting you exhausted or pushing you to the point of discomfort. A study published in the National Library of Medicine demonstrated that yoga intervention is effective in managing insomnia and other sleep problems (Wang et al. 2020).

While the list of yoga benefits is endless, you may end up not reaping any or even worsening your situation.

Wondering why?

How you perform the sequences matters the most than any other thing. Failing to get it right may cost you. That's why in this book we present to you step-by-step instructions on how to correctly perform the most impactful chair yoga sequences.

How to Use This Book

Regardless of where you decide to start reading this book, we recommend reading through the following paragraphs which highlight the principles of yoga, precautions, and what you need to get started with your chair yoga programs. We also encourage you to read through chapter 1 "Breathing Techniques" and ensure that you've grasped the breathing concepts and that you can control your breathing before you begin practicing yoga. Most poses are accompanied by illustrations to help you visualize the written instructions.

The programs in this book are perfect for:

- Beginners looking for a low-risk, low-stakes way to try yoga for the first time
- People with osteoarthritis of the hands, knees, and hips
- Seniors looking for exercise that is easy on the joints and known to reduce aches and pains
- Individuals who because of injury or limitations in mobility want to avoid standing poses and/or floor poses
- Anyone who is sedentary and wants chair exercises to offset the negative effects of prolonged sitting
- Anyone that can benefit from a convenient and affordable chair yoga program
- Yoga teachers looking for creative moves and novel sequences to add to their chair yoga repertoire

We've divided the yoga practice programs into the following categories:

- Breathing techniques
- Warm-up exercises
- Specialized Introductory Program for Absolute Beginners
- Dedicated Intermediate Program

- Exclusive Advanced Program

- Beginner program for osteoarthritis of the hands, knees, and hips

- Intermediate program for osteoarthritis of the hands, knees, and hip

Each of the above programs has a range of different poses/ sequences that best suit people with the specified levels and program descriptions. This is to help make your chair yoga practice comfortable, safe, and fulfilling as possible while considering any physical limitations you might experience. Each sequence takes 10 minutes after the warm-up, so you can follow each or choose as your schedule allows.

Principles of YOGA

Just like any other physical exercise, yoga has guiding principles that you need to follow to maximize your performance and reap the most out of the benefits that yoga practice brings. The following principles apply to all types of yoga including chair yoga.

- **Proper Breathing:** Breathing is key in yoga. We emphasize a lot on correct breathing because it helps your body stay wired to your mind and concentrated on the present. Be mindful of your yoga breathing techniques and follow the breath cues in the instructions to ensure that you're getting the most out of your practice.

- **Proper Body Form and Exercise:** Performing your yoga practice in proper form and the right way helps avoid injuries. Perform your yoga exercises slowly, gently, and with complete awareness.

- **Proper Relaxation:** Work towards achieving a complete relaxation of the body and mind. Do whatever it takes to release all the tension from your muscles and brain. The best way to achieve relaxation is to begin with a breathing technique and warm-up exercises (discussed in Chapters One and Two) that will help you feel relaxed before the actual yoga practice.

- **Positive Thinking and Meditation:** Yoga requires self-motivation, desire, and positive vibes. Thinking positively will make you content. Be thankful and proud of what you have, who you are, and what you can achieve.

- **Proper Nutrition:** Exercise and nutrition are like pillars that make up a structure such that if you overlook or pull down one of them, the entire structure collapses. Without a proper diet, you won't benefit much from yoga practice. So you need to be mindful of the calories you consume too.

Precautions

As much as chair yoga is the safest and most gentle road to take towards achieving your fitness goals, never jump into it without your doctor's advice and the "go ahead" to do so. Ask your doctor about the exercises you should and should not do. Yoga exercises and poses are sometimes challenging; however, you shouldn't feel pain when practicing any posture. "Listen" to your body, in case you feel any pain in a pose, stop immediately. Always work within a pain-free range of motion. In yoga, there are several ways to achieve the same objective. That's why you will find in this book a couple of poses that stretch the same muscle and different poses for people with different activity levels. So always feel free to skip a pose and move to what you feel is easier for you or best suits your activity level and condition.

Pay special attention to the following health issues:

- **Osteoporosis:** Always make the movements in a slow manner and in complete awareness to lubricate and create space in your joints. In case of a pose that involves twisting, always choose the gentlest variation and NEVER force yourself into a twisted position using your hands. When performing a pose that involves forward bending from the waist, move from the hip joint without rounding your back, and don't go past 45 degrees. Above all, always avoid bouncing and impact.

- **High or low blood pressure:** For poses that involve moving the head and/or chest up or down, move slowly and with awareness to allow the body to adapt to the change.

- **Spinal arthritis/bone degeneration and spurs:** Always keep the head straight when performing a posture that involves bending backward. Don't let your head fall at the back.

What You Need to Get Started

You don't need any fancy equipment to perform chair yoga. You just need a chair, your breath, your desire, and your body. To make yourself more comfortable and stable while you practice your chair yoga, consider the following:

CLOTHING

Wear loose and comfortable clothes that you can move in easily. Ensure you are warm enough. Don't wear shoes, perform all your chair yoga postures on bare feet.

YOGA MAT

You may place a yoga mat under your chair to help prevent it from sliding on the floor and to cushion your feet to prevent friction.

TYPE OF CHAIR

You need a sturdy, solid, and armless chair that will stick in the same position as you move. You may also have any other yoga props like foam blocks, a bolster, or blankets that may provide comfortable support to your feet and sitz bones.

Chapter One:
Breathing Techniques (Pranayama)

The emphasis on breathing is what makes yoga magical and unique from other physical activities. Otherwise, it would be merely stretching and calisthenics. Proper breathing is the main principle of yoga; it is one of the most valuable tools for changing the state of your mind. It helps you feel relaxed and maintain focus, heat in the body, and good circulation as well as cooling you down when overheated. As opposed to most aerobic exercises where you have to breathe through your mouth to help cool your body, most yoga breathing is usually through your nostril helping you maintain heat in the body.

The breathing technique is one of the easiest movements to incorporate and implement in your daily routine. Every yoga posture begins with breathing. The breathing practice in yoga is what we refer to as *pranayama* which means "control of the breath". In this chapter, you will find a series of different breathing techniques you can easily incorporate into your routine to help heat up or cool down your body as well as reap other benefits while you practice your chair yoga poses. Just take your time to learn how to perform each of the techniques correctly and you will see changes instantly.

Alternate Nostril Breathing (Nadi Shodhana)

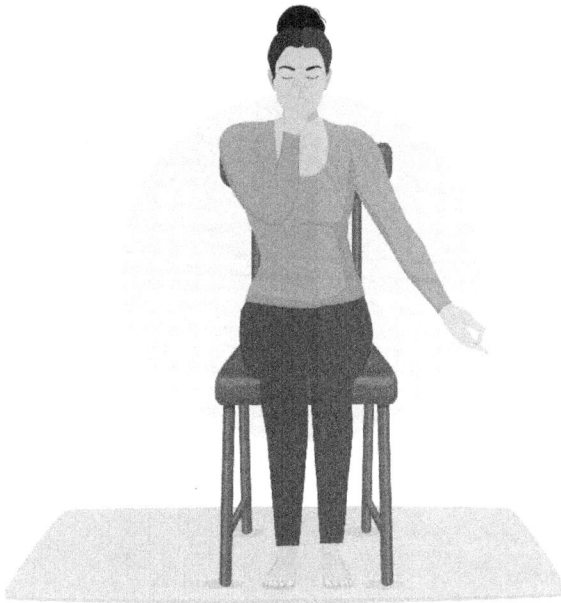

Paying attention to your breath quality and tracking its flow through your nostrils is one of the fastest ways to collect and calm yourself. This breathing technique calms you down immediately whenever you feel anxious or agitated. It also improves sleep and nasal respiration and boosts thinking.

Step-by-Step Instructions

- Sit up tall and comfortable in the chair with your spine erect and relaxed, feet planted firmly on the floor at about hip-width apart, and breathe in and out slowly through both nostrils to make yourself more comfortable.

- Place your right thumb on your right nostril and your ring finger or right forefinger on the left nostril maintaining light contact with them throughout. Close your right nostril by pressing it gently with the thumb and inhale through the left nostril.

- Release your thumb and close your left nostril by gently pressing it with your right forefinger or ring finger and breathe out through your left nostril.

- Repeat alternating between your left and right nostrils.

Ocean Breath (Ujjayi Pranayama)

This yoga breathing technique is used when flowing and holding through postures. It helps you stay alert, relaxed, and energized.

Step-by-Step Instructions

- Sit up tall and comfortable in the chair with your feet flat on the ground.

- Rest your hands on your knees with palms facing upwards and thumbs and forefingers interlaced.

- Breathe in slightly deeper than normal through your nose, then breathe out with your mouth open and make a silent extended "haaaaah" sound. Repeat this twice.

- Now try to make a similar sound on both the inhalation and exhalation with your mouth closed and breathing through the nose. To achieve this, you will need to constrict your throat gently, closing off its back as you inhale.

Cleansing Breath (Kapalbhati)

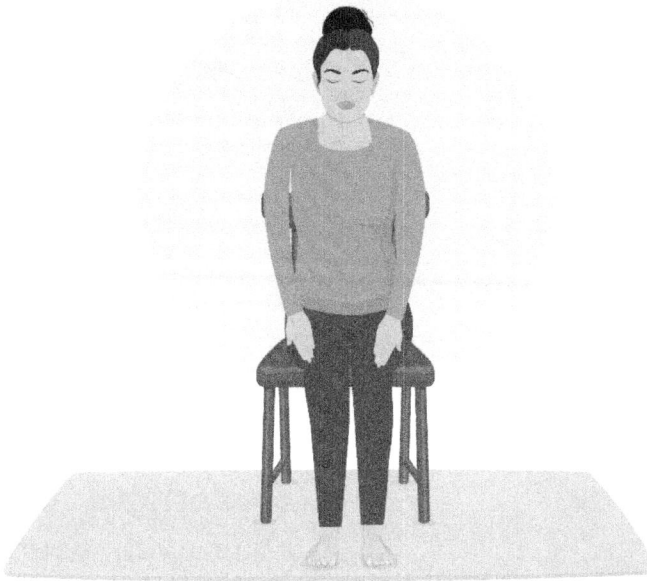

Kapalbhati Pranayama also known as "Skull Shining" is a famous yoga breathing technique among yogis for clearing the mind. This breathing technique is an excellent way to remove "cobwebs" in your mind and lungs and increase your concentration level. Besides, it helps work your core and lower abs, relieve stress, increase metabolism and boost energy.

Step-by-Step Instructions

- Sit up tall in the chair leaving some space behind you so that you are not leaning on it.

- Plant your feet flat and firmly on the floor with your hands hanging by your sides

- Rest your hands on your thighs just above the knees with palms facing up.

- Take a deep full breath in through your nose, then breathe out all the air as you pull your navel and the belly back towards the spine. Next, take a partial breath in and exhale quickly through the nose relaxing the navel and the abdomen. You may pump at a pace of your choice. Just ensure that the breath is continuous but the "breathe ins" are very subtle and small. Perform as many pumps as you can. Start smaller and build your way up.

- On the last pump, stop and take a full breath in and a full breath out.

Bellows Breath (Bhastrika)

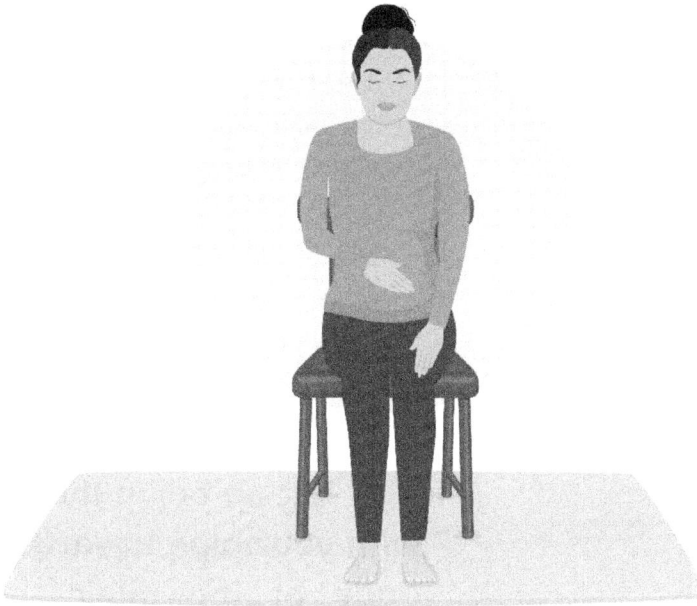

This type of yogic breathing helps energize and awaken your entire body. It also helps clear your mind, relieves stress from the brain, builds abdominal strength, increases your lung capacity, boosts digestion, and increases metabolism.

Step-by-Step Instructions

- Sit up tall in the chair with your hips towards the edge of the chair, back straight, your feet planted firmly on the floor at a hip-width apart.

- Place one hand on your belly and keep the other one resting on your thigh.

- Take a short forceful breath in followed by a short, sharp breath out.

- Do it over and over again for about one minute

- On the last pump, take a break before you repeat the pumping

Just as the name suggests, Kumbhaka Pranayama is a breathing technique that involves holding the breath after inhaling or exhaling. Breath retention helps increase pressure in your lungs giving them time to fully expand, increasing their capacity. This increases the flow of oxygenated blood to the heart, brain, and muscles.

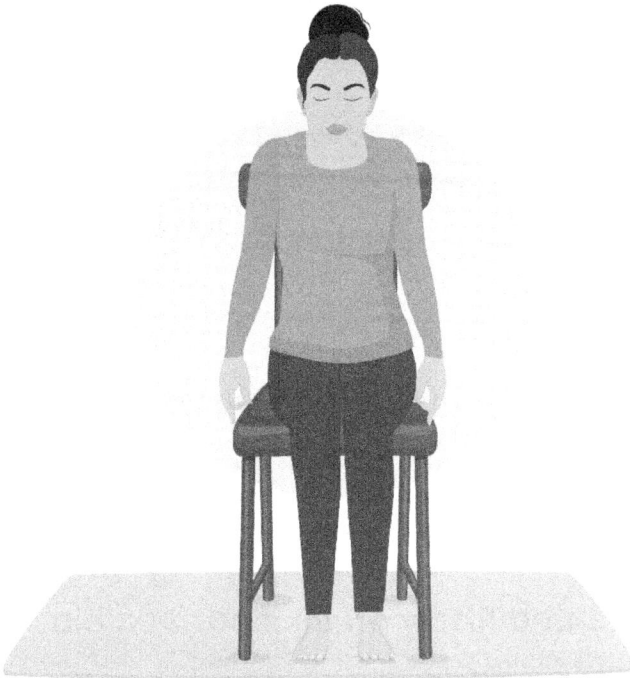

Step-by-Step Instructions

- Sit up tall in the chair with your hips towards the edge of the chair, back straight, your feet planted firmly on the floor at a hip-width apart.

- Take a deep, full breath in and try to picture it circulating in your heart. Lower your head down bringing your chin close to your chest as you inflate your lungs. Hold your breath until you feel you can no longer do it, then exhale all the air out.

- Once all the air is completely out, hold empty for as long as you can before inflating your lungs again.

Cooling Breath (Sitali)

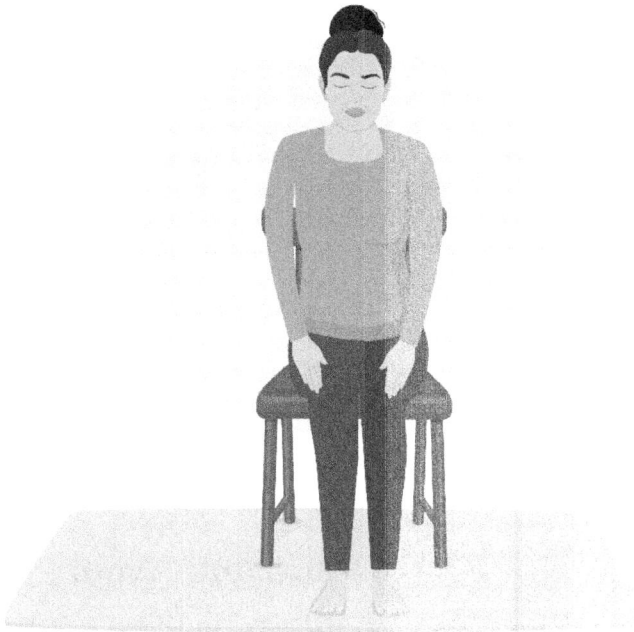

Sithali helps cool down and calm your body. Our bodies may become overheated due to changes in our external and internal temperatures, or after performing a yoga session or any other workout. Practicing this breathing technique will help you cool down when you feel overheated.

Step-by-Step Instruction

- Sit up tall in the chair with your hips towards the edge of the chair, back straight, your feet planted firmly on the floor at a hip-width apart.

- Place your palms face-down on your thighs.

- Take deep breaths in and out twice or thrice through your nose to prepare for this pranayama.

- Curl the sides of your tongue inwards towards the center to roll it into a tube-like shape. If you can't roll your tongue, purse your lips to make a small "o" shape with your mouth.

- Inhale slowly through the tube if you roll your tongue or channel the air through the "o" shaped opening if your lips are pursed.

- Close your mouth and breathe out slowly through your nose.

- Repeat until you feel the maximum cooling effect

Hissing Teeth Breath (Sitkari)

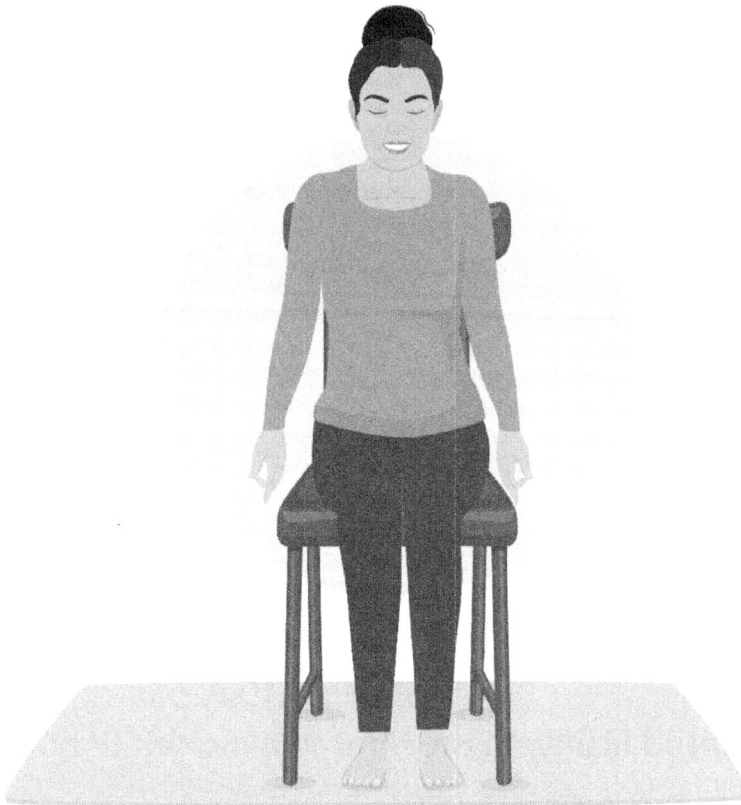

This is also another cooling breath technique that helps refresh the body and mind.

Step-by-Step Instruction

- Sit up tall in the chair with your hips towards the edge of the chair, back straight, your feet planted firmly on the floor at a hip-width apart.

- Take a few natural breaths in and out to center yourself.

- With your lips open, close your teeth by bringing your lower and upper teeth together and inhale through them producing a soft hissing sound.

- Release the teeth and close your mouth as you breathe out through the nose

- Repeat until you feel a nice cooling effect that eases your body and mind.

Chapter Two: Warm-Up Exercises

Warm-ups are important when performing any physical activity, including yoga. They help lubricate your joints, strengthen your muscles and stretch your body preparing it for efficient and effective performance without sustaining injuries. Chair yoga warm-up exercises also increase blood flow to your muscles preparing them for more challenging and longer-held postures.

Besides, chair yoga warm-up will help you link your breath to the exercise and prepare your mind to be calm and focused, preventing you from distractions. So, always begin all sessions with 5 – 10 minutes of gentle warm-ups. Going right away to the yoga postures without warming up your body increases your risks of injuries and makes you perform poorly. It is like trying to start an old car on a freezing winter morning. It is probably going to stutter and sputter until the engine finally dies.

In this chapter, I will share with you **the most productive, but gentle chair yoga warm-up exercises.** Try to always begin each of your chair yoga sessions with this routine, and you will see how your body unwinds in a much calmer, focused, and energized way. Try to stay in a seated position the entire time. Flow at a pace of your choice. It can be slow or faster. As you perform the moves, ensure that your body and your breath are connected. Pay attention to your breathing and the movement; they should flow at the same pace. Ensure that there are completely no sources of distraction. Put your gadgets (phone, laptop, tablets, etc.) on silent mode or keep them switched off.

Chair Mountain Pose (Chair Tadasana)

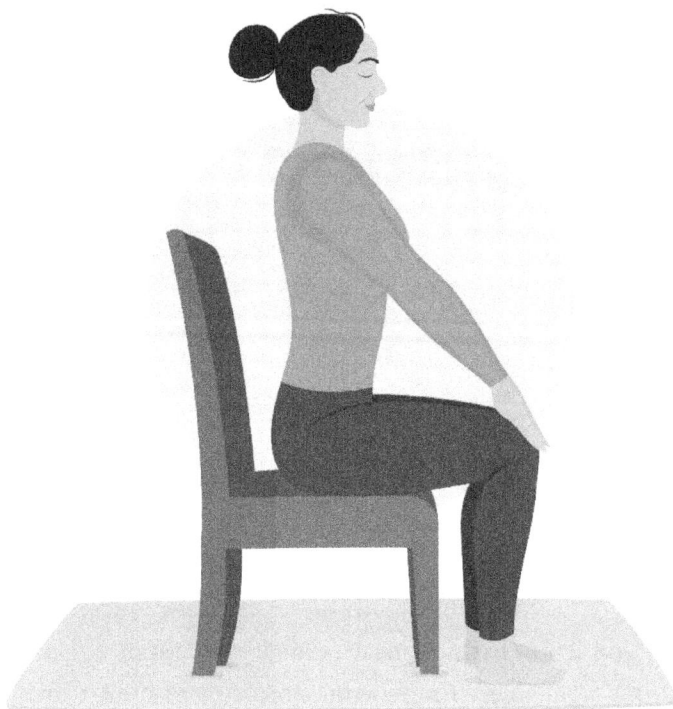

This chair yoga warm-up exercise helps calm your body and mind, making you feel more grounded and ready to perform other sequences. It warms up your back muscles, heart, and shoulder muscles.

Step-by-Step Instruction

- Begin by sitting up tall in your chair, leaving some space behind you.

- Keep your spine lengthened, shoulders neutral with chest raised, and engage your abdominal muscles.

- Plant your feet flat and firmly on the floor at a hip distance apart with toes pointed straight ahead.

- Keep your limbs and face relaxed

- Place your palms flat on top of your upper thighs

- Close your eyes and take 10-15 complete deep breaths in and out through your nose.

- Slowly and gently open your eyes and release your hands down by your sides to come out of the pose.

Seated Neck Rolls (Kantasanchalana)

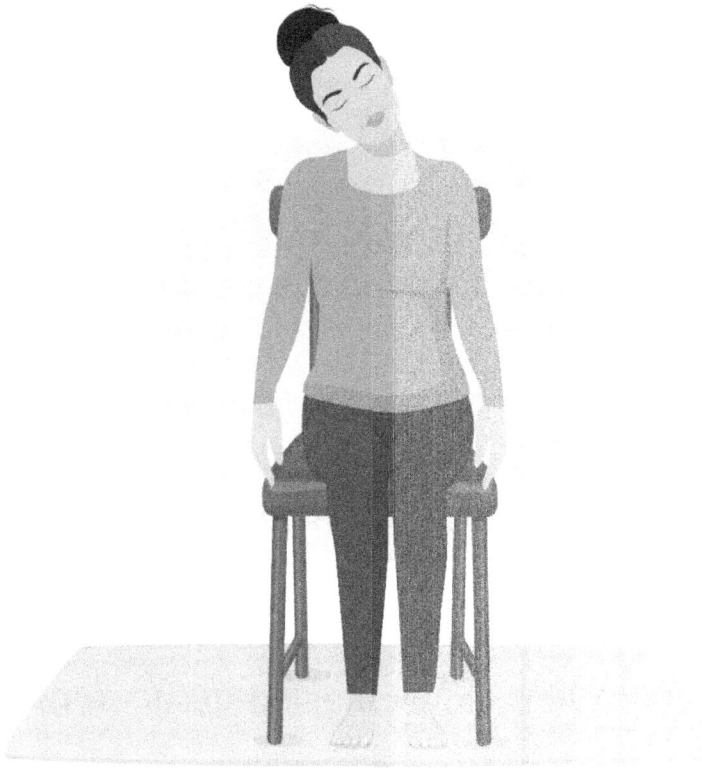

If you spend a lot of time sitting, neck rolls are the best warm-up for your chair yoga sequences. It helps release tension from your neck muscles and lubricates your neck joint.

Step-by-Step Instructions

- Sit up tall towards the edge of the chair, lengthen through your spine, and keep your abdominal muscles engaged, shoulders neutral with chest raised.

- Plant your feet flat and firm on the floor at a hip distance apart with toes pointed straight ahead.

- Place your palms face-down on top of your upper thighs and relax your face and limbs

- Take a deep breath in and out through your nose while dropping your chin towards your chest. This is the starting position.

- Maintaining your natural breathing pattern, rotate your head around gently by bringing your left ear towards your left shoulder.

- Keep the rotation going by bringing your head around to the back, gazing up to the ceiling, and keeping the back neck length as long as possible.

- Rotate your head around as gently as possible bringing your right ear towards your right shoulder.

- Roll your head down towards the ground with your chin toward your chest to bring it back to the starting position.

- Repeat steps 4 to 7 five to ten times.

- Repeat the rotations five to time times moving in the opposite direction.

- Bring your head back up gently facing forward after performing your final rotation.

Chair Cat-Cow Stretch (Chair Marjaryasana Bitilasana)

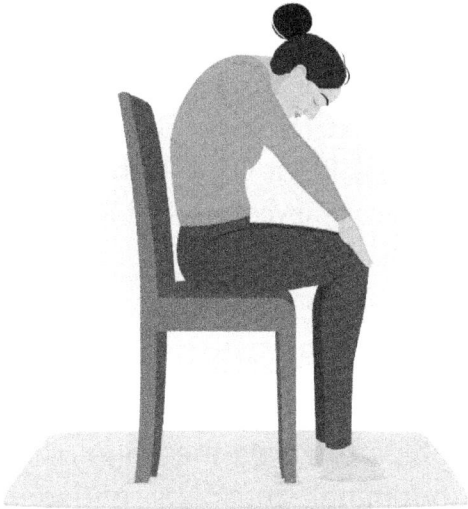

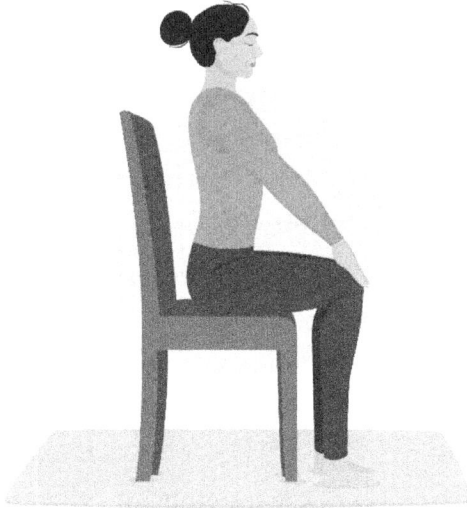

Cat/cow stretch warms up your entire spine, back, shoulders, abdominals, hips, and pelvic floor muscles. It helps an achy back which is very common among older adults. It is good to begin your chair yoga practice with this warm-up because it helps expand your breath, perk up and open your entire body.

Step-by-Step Instructions

- Sit up tall at the edge of the chair, with the spine long, abdominal muscles engaged, shoulders neutral and chest raised.

- Plant your feet flat and firm on the floor at a hip distance apart with toes pointed straight forward.

- Place your palms face-down just above your knees

- When breathing in, bring your chest outward while sticking your hips out behind you.

- Gaze at the ceiling keeping your shoulder blades gently squeezed together.

- Breathe out as you round your chest and spine, scooping your belly inwards, curling under your tailbone as you drop your jawline towards your chest, letting your shoulders approach your ears.

- Repeat for a series of 5-10 cycles.

Pelvic Tilts/Circles

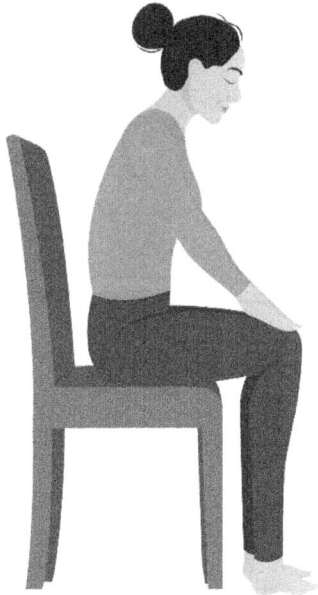

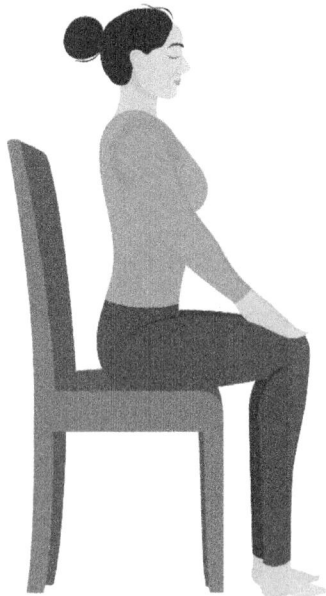

It is always important to warm up your pelvis and lower abs before starting your yoga practice. This is because your pelvic floor region forms the base of your spine and upper body when seated. Tapping into it is a great way to access your organic energy and stay steady all day long. Pelvic circles warm up your spine and lower back, loosen up your lower body and work your pelvic floor and abdominal muscles.

Step-by-Step Instruction

- Sit up tall with your hips towards the edge of the chair, spine long, abdominal muscles engaged, shoulders neutral and chest raised.

- Plant your feet flat and firm on the floor at a hip distance apart with toes pointed straight forward.

- Place your palms face-down on your knees and try to imagine having a marble on your navel and you want it rolled down through your inner thighs.

- Pull your navel inwards imagining you are trying to bring the marble back up in front of your belly towards your navel as you tip your sit bones. Ensure that you isolate just your pelvis. Don't tense your shoulders or arch your upper back.

- Keep rounding and arching your tailbone for about 8 cycles.

- Maintaining the same position, make circles in both clockwise and anticlockwise directions with your pelvis five times for each direction.

Foot and Ankle Stretch

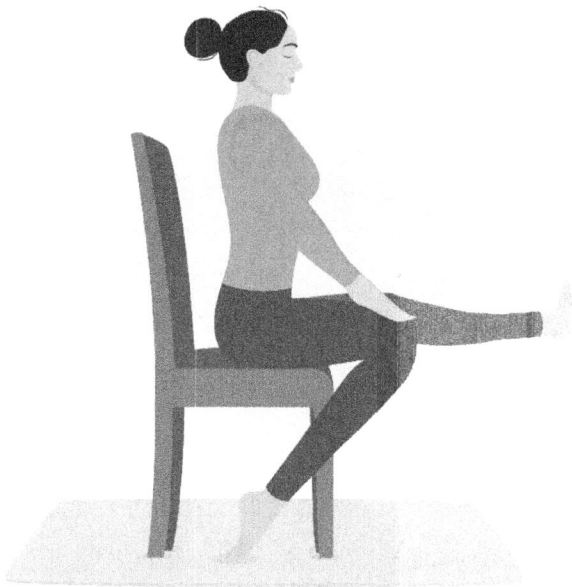

This move helps warm up your ankles, feet, and legs. It also helps lubricate your limb joints increasing their mobility. Foot and ankle stretch makes your feet and ankle muscles more flexible and helps you prevent pain during long walks.

Step-by-Step Instruction

- Begin by sitting up tall in your chair, leaving some space behind you.

- Keep your spine lengthened, shoulders neutral with chest raised, and engage your abdominal muscles.

- Plant your feet flat and firmly on the floor at a hip distance apart with toes pointed straight ahead.

- Place your palms face down on top of your upper thighs and relax your face and limbs

- Extend your left leg straight out in front of you, place your heel on the floor and flex your foot.

- Point your toes towards the ground; ensure that you feel a gentle stretch in the top of your foot

- Keep flexing and pointing your toes towards the floor 5 to 10 times and then bring your left leg back next to the right leg in a gentle manner.

- Repeat steps 4 to 6 with your right leg.

- Do it 5-10 times alternating the legs.

Seated Shoulder Rolls

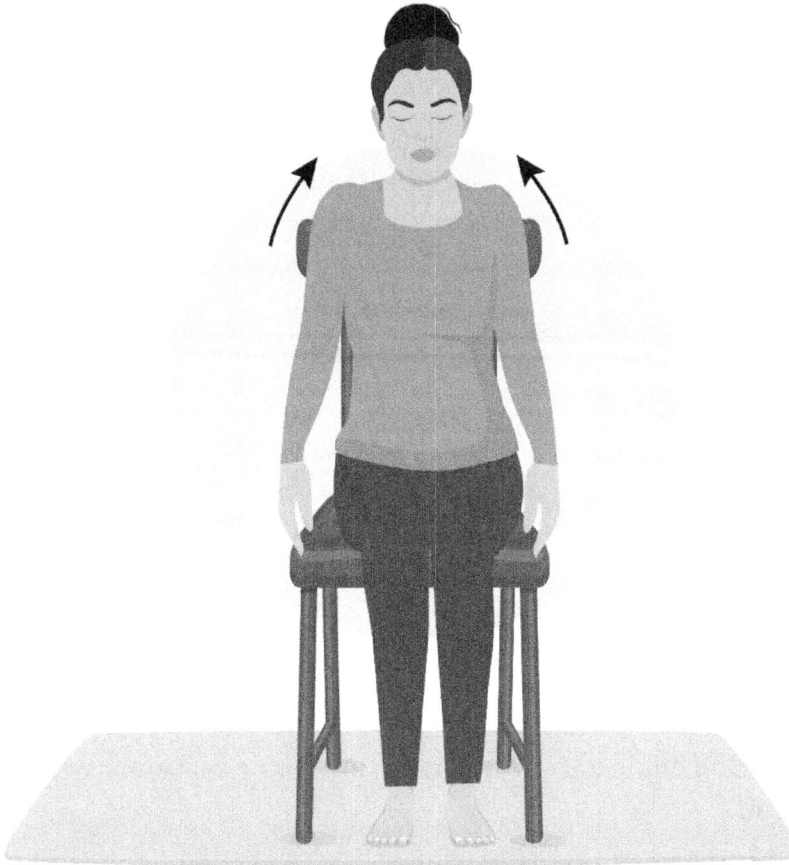

Shoulder rolls help warm up your neck, shoulders, and upper back. They are good for loosening your muscles and lubricating your shoulder joints thus increasing their mobility.

Step-by-Step Instructions

- **Sit upright in the chair so that your back isn't leaning on the chair**

- **Keep your feet flat and firmly planted on the floor at a hip distance apart with your palms on your thighs.**

- Take a deep breath in through your nose, lifting both shoulders towards your ears.

- On a breath out, slowly and gently roll both shoulders back and down in a circular motion.

- Continue rolling your shoulders back and down in a smooth and gentle, continuous motion for 5 to 10 rotations.

- Repeat steps 3 and 4 in the alternate direction for 5-10 rotations

Seated Side Bend Pose

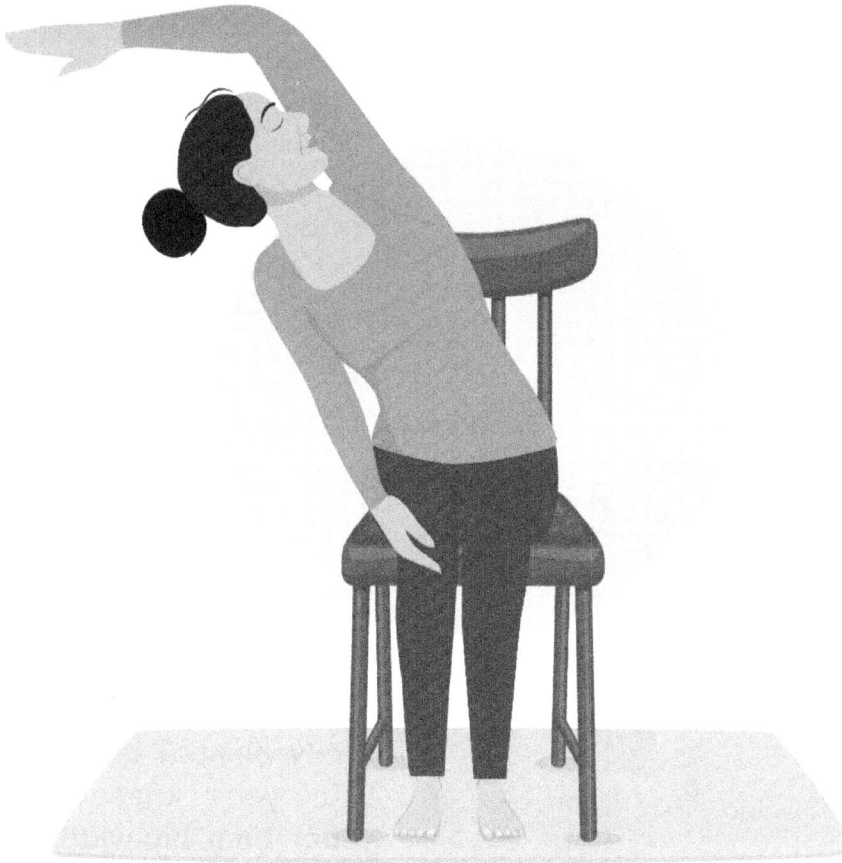

This pose stretches the neck, shoulders, back, arms and obliques. It is a good warm-up exercise for gaining joint mobility and flexibility in your arms, shoulders, and upper body muscles.

Step-by-Step Instruction

- Sit up tall in the chair so that your back isn't leaning on it

- Keep your feet flat and firmly planted on the floor at a hip distance apart with your palms on your thighs.

- Remaining firmly seated on the chair with both your shin bones planted on it, place your right palm face-down on your left thigh and reach your left hand up and over to the left facing forward and tilting your torso over slightly to the right.

- Hold the pose for a few seconds (for one deep and complete breath). You should feel the stretch on the left side of the torso.

- Release yourself slowly back to a neutral position with your spine upright and arms down by your sides.

- Switch to the opposite side and repeat.

Sun Salutations

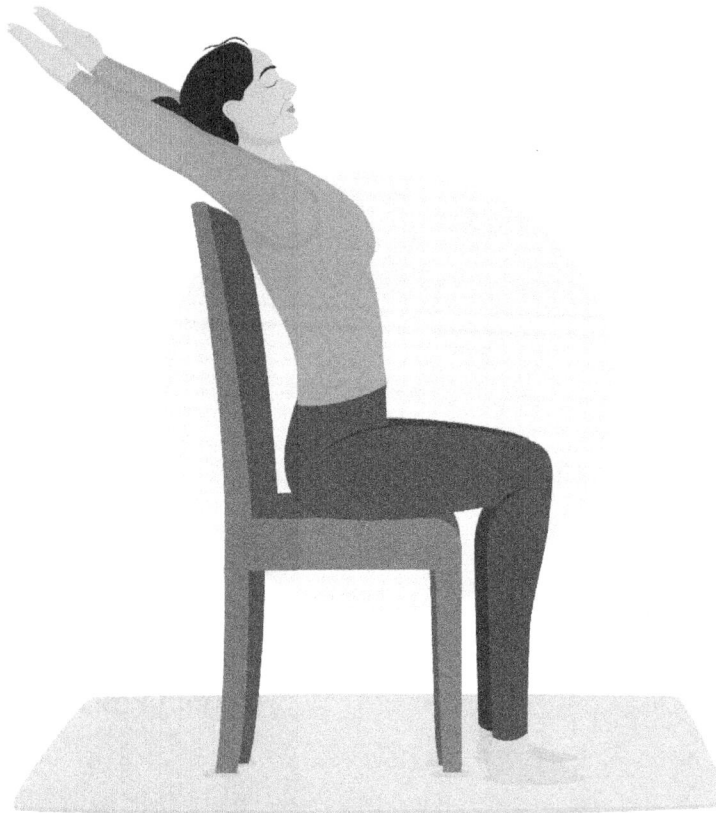

Performing sun salutations enhances better blood circulation, breath expansion, and increased flexibility. They bring warmth and heat into our bodies releasing the tension in our shoulders, head, and neck. The following sun salutation sequence is a great way to warm up.

Step-by-Step Instructions

- Sit up in the chair leaving some space behind you

- Keep your feet flat and firmly planted on the floor with your knees slightly wider than hip-width apart and palms face-down on top of your thighs.

- On a breath in, sweep your hands outwards to your sides and then lift them overhead.

- On a breath out, slowly and gently lower your hand back to the thighs leaning forward while flattening your back.

- Fold over as you breathe in and out until your hands rest on your shins or floor.

- Breathe in and come back to the starting position with a flat back and hands resting on your thighs then breathe out.

- Repeat steps 3 to 5 for 5 -10 times.

Marching Flow

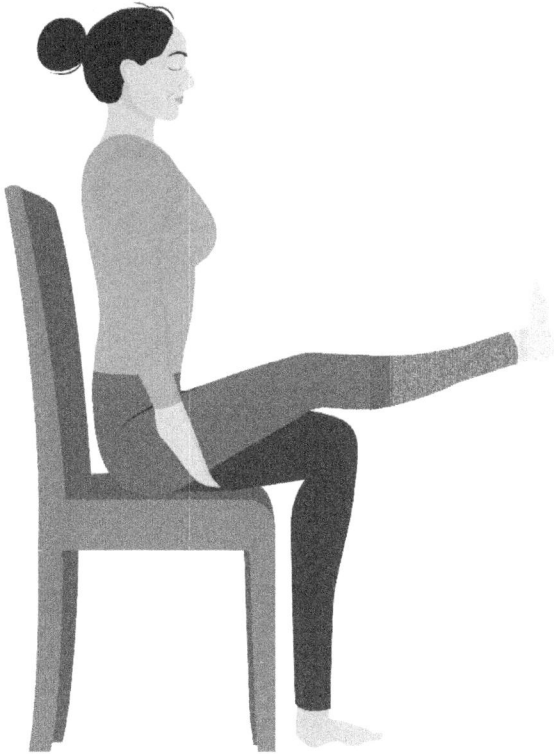

Most seniors spent most of their time seated. Staying seated for a prolonged period makes you feel restricted and tied up in your hips and lower back. The matching flow gets your legs moving, boosting metabolism and working them out. Most yoga exercises concentrate more on large muscle groups and this pose also gets our lower half warmed up. It works on your core, external rotators, quadriceps, and inner thighs.

Step-by-Step Instruction

- Sit tall in the chair, with your back straight leaving some space behind you so that your back isn't leaning on it.

- Keep your feet flat and firmly planted on the floor at a hip distance apart with your palms on your thighs.

- Breathe in as you straighten your right leg out in front of you; ensure to engage your quadriceps and lengthen behind your knee.

- Breathe out and bend your knee to open your right hip as you rest the right outer ankle on your left knee (you may be required to use your hand to help place the foot on your knee and open the leg).

- Breathe in and slowly and gently extend the leg back forward, then breathe out and gently lower the foot and put it on the floor.

- Repeat the sequence alternating the legs.

Knee Swings

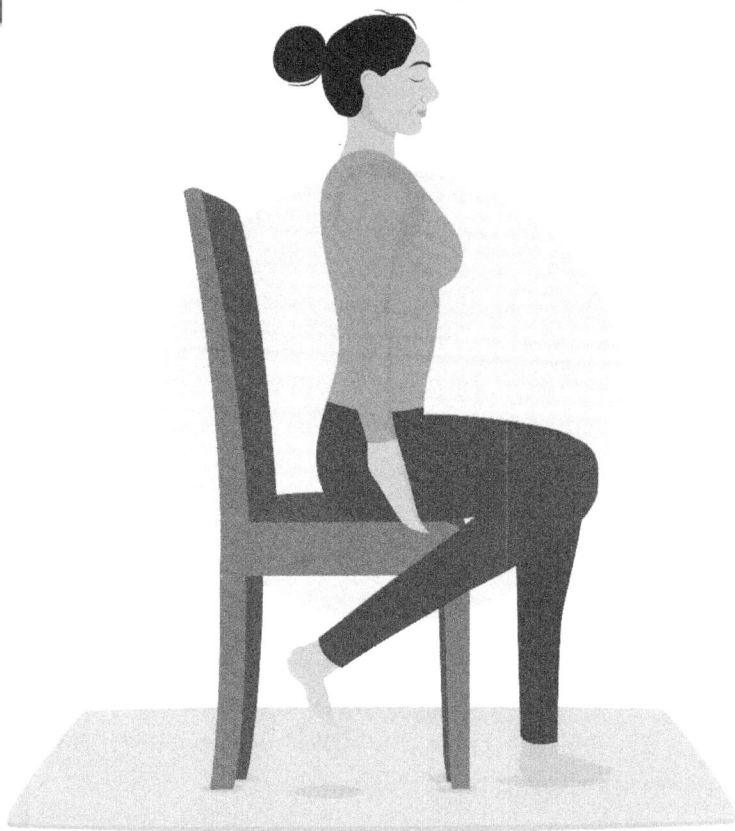

This is among the few poses that are done quickly. If you can't reach under your knee with your back straight, then just sit back in the chair and do the kicks swinging back and forth at a speed you are comfortable with. This warm-up exercise helps lubricate the knee joint thus increasing mobility and range of motion in the knees.

Step-by-Step Instructions

- Sit up tall in the chair leaving some space behind you.

- Keep your back straight, shoulders neutral, and engage your abdominal muscles

- Plant your feet flat and firmly on the floor at a hip distance apart with toes pointed straight ahead and arms hanging by your sides.

- Clasp both hands under your right knee while maintaining a straight back.

- While holding your knee, begin kicking your leg out back and forth

- Repeat alternating the legs.

Chapter Three:
Our Specialized Introductory Program
for Absolute Beginners

In this chapter, you will find our specialized introductory program meant for absolute beginners. The program includes a sequence of chair yoga poses that are simple and easy to follow. They are the best way to start your chair yoga journey and gradually increase your body strength, flexibility, stability, and mobility while being very kind and gentle to yourself.

You can perform these exercises as a stand-alone routine or in a combination with the warm-up sequence from the previous chapter. But is it important to prepare your mind and breathing system to increase your concentration level during the exercise. So we will start with a breathing exercise to help keep your nose ready for nasal respiration and strengthen your lungs. Let's begin!

Breathing Exercise

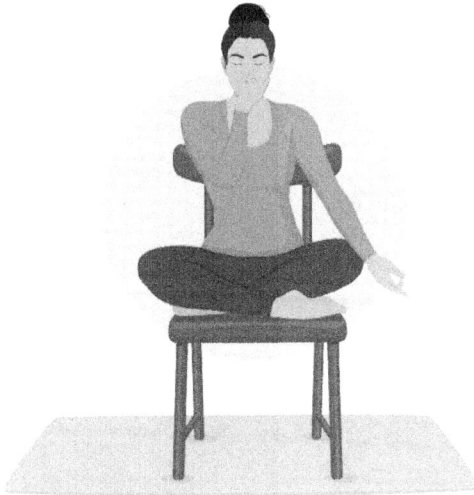

At this level, alternate nostril breathing (Nadi Shodhana) will do you good. As you already know, the breathing technique helps calm you down and improve nasal respiration. So by starting with this breathing exercise, you will be able to collect and calm yourself if you feel anxious or agitated before getting started with the actual yoga moves. Besides, yoga requires you to breathe through your nose throughout. Therefore, this breathing technique will prepare your nostrils.

Step-by-Step Instructions

- Start from the meditation sitting position above.
- Place your right thumb on your right nostril and your ring finger or right forefinger on the left nostril. Maintain light contact with them throughout the breathing exercise.
- Close your right nostril by pressing it gently with the thumb and inhale through the left nostril.
- Release your thumb and close your left nostril by gently pressing it with your right forefinger or ring finger and breathe out through your right nostril.
- Keep your left nostril closed and breathe in through your right nostril
- Release your forefinger or ring finger on your left nose and close your right nose by gently pressing your right thumb and breathe out through your left nostril.
- This makes up one round.
- Do it for two rounds

Warm Up Your Body

To warm up your body, perform the sequence of warm-up exercises discussed in the previous chapter. You may select a few of the exercises that you feel are easier for you. Remember, this is not mandatory. As mentioned earlier, you can perform these exercises as a standalone routine because they also include warm-up exercises.

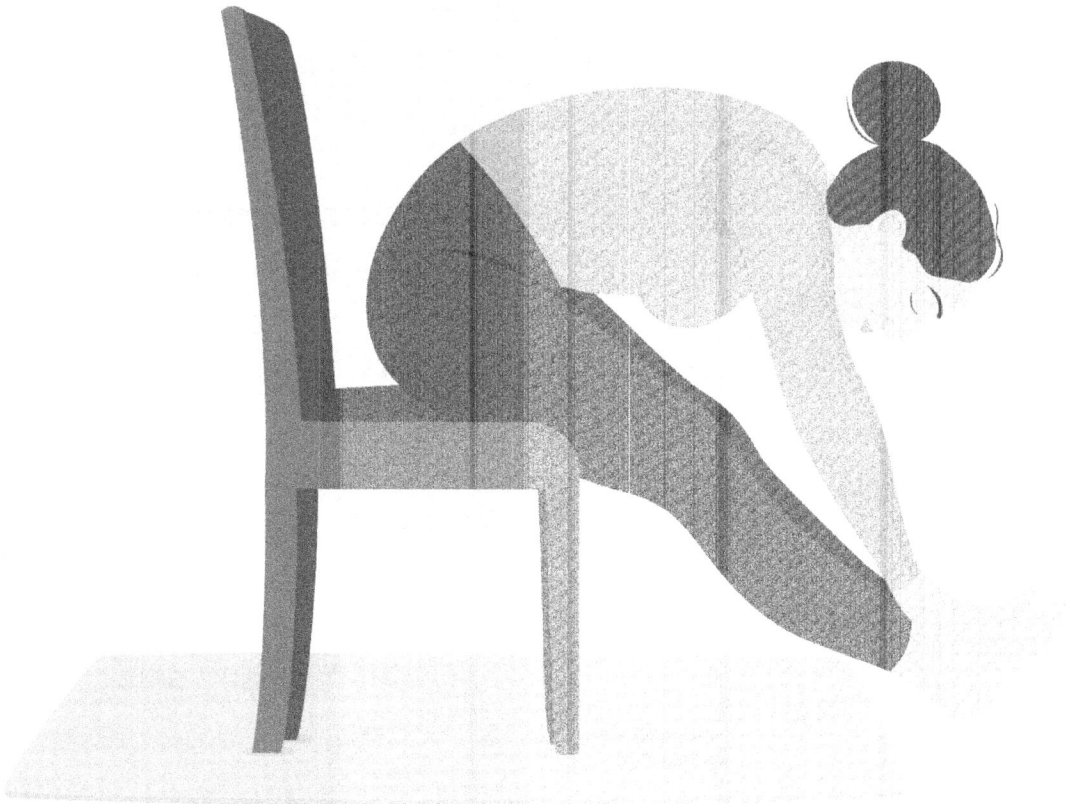

Looking Left and Right

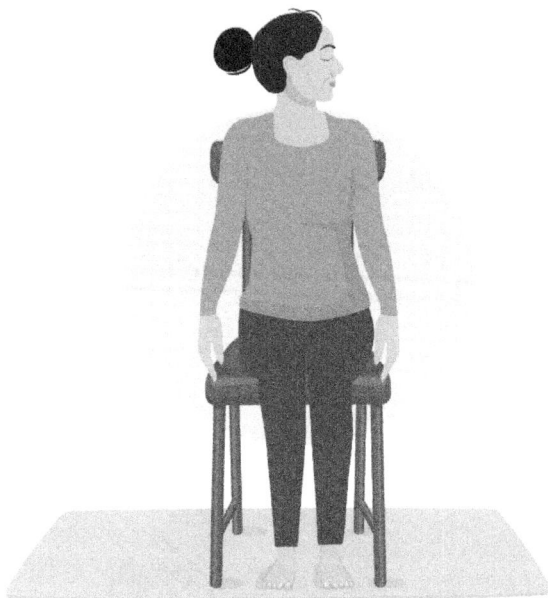

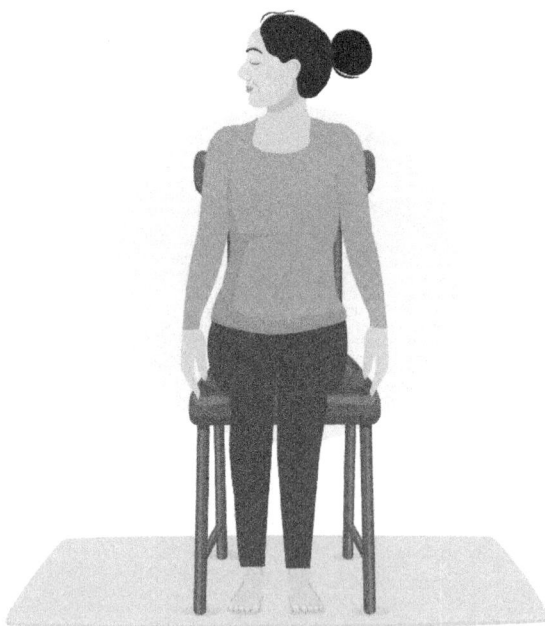

This move works out and stretches the muscles surrounding your neck. It helps improve the flexibility and mobility of your neck.

Step-by-Step Instructions

- Sit up tall and comfortable at the edge of the chair with your spine erect and relaxed, feet flat on the floor at about hip-width apart.

- Rest your hands on your upper thighs just above your knees and take a deep breath in through your nose and slowly exhale.

- Turn your head gently to the left, and pause for a few deep breaths. Ensure that you move as far as you can without experiencing any discomfort.

- Bring your head back slowly and gently, turning it to the right.

- Repeat for both sides.

Assisted Neck Stretch

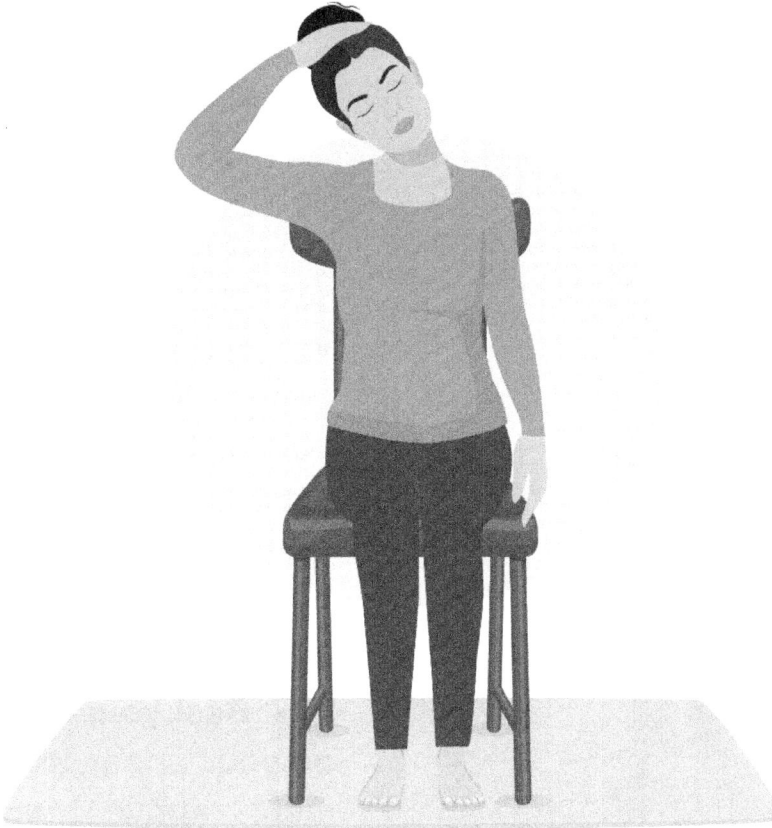

This pose works out your neck and shoulder muscles. It helps gain flexibility and joint mobility in neck and shoulder muscles and joints. It also helps relieve stress and tension.

Step-by-Step Instructions

- Sit up tall and comfortable towards the edge of the chair with your spine erect and relaxed, feet planted firmly on the floor at about hip-width apart.

- Rest your hands on your upper thighs just above your knees and take a deep breath in through your nose and slowly exhale.

- Tilt your head gently towards the right, maintaining even shoulders.

- Using your right hand, lightly wrap the top of your head and tilt it, over-stretching the left side of your neck. Ensure not to pull it with force.

- Hold there for 5-10 deep inhales and exhales

- Release your hand slowly and bring your head back to return to the starting position

- Repeat on the opposite side.

Up-Down, Right-Left (Eye movement)

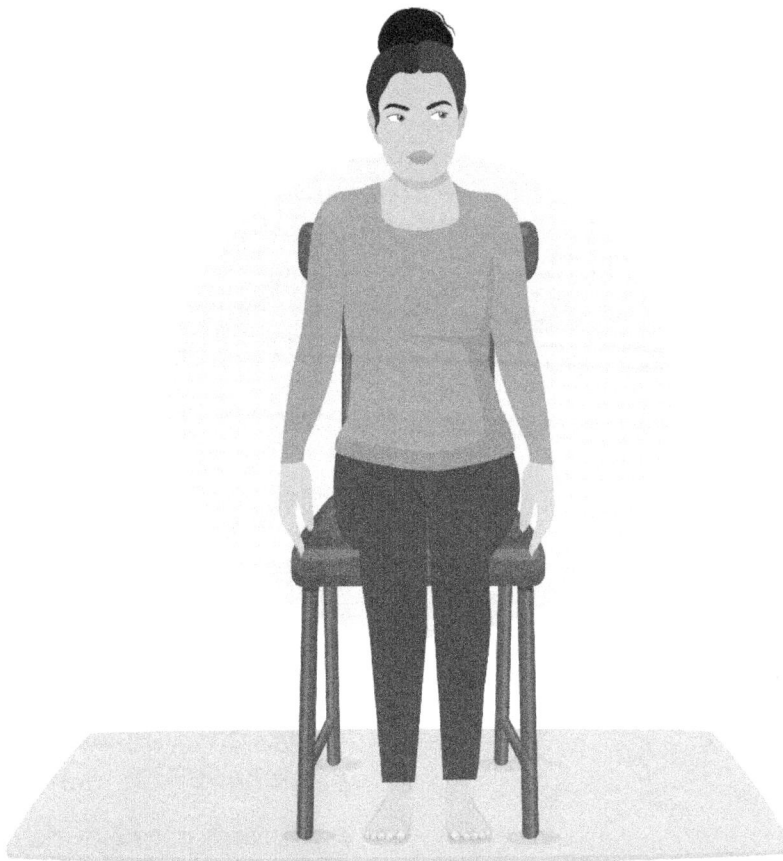

This move strengthens the extraocular muscles of the eyes and helps reduce tension.

Step-by-Step-Instructions

- Sit up tall and comfortable at the edge of the chair with your spine erect and relaxed, feet flat on the floor at about hip-width apart.

- Rest your hands on your upper thighs just above your knees and take a deep breath in through your nose and slowly exhale. Ensure that your head and torso are still.

- Move your eyes up and down about 3-5 times.

- Close your eyes and take a deep breath in and out.

- Move your eyes to the left and look to the right 3-5 times

- Close your eyes and take a deep breath in and out.

- Repeat.

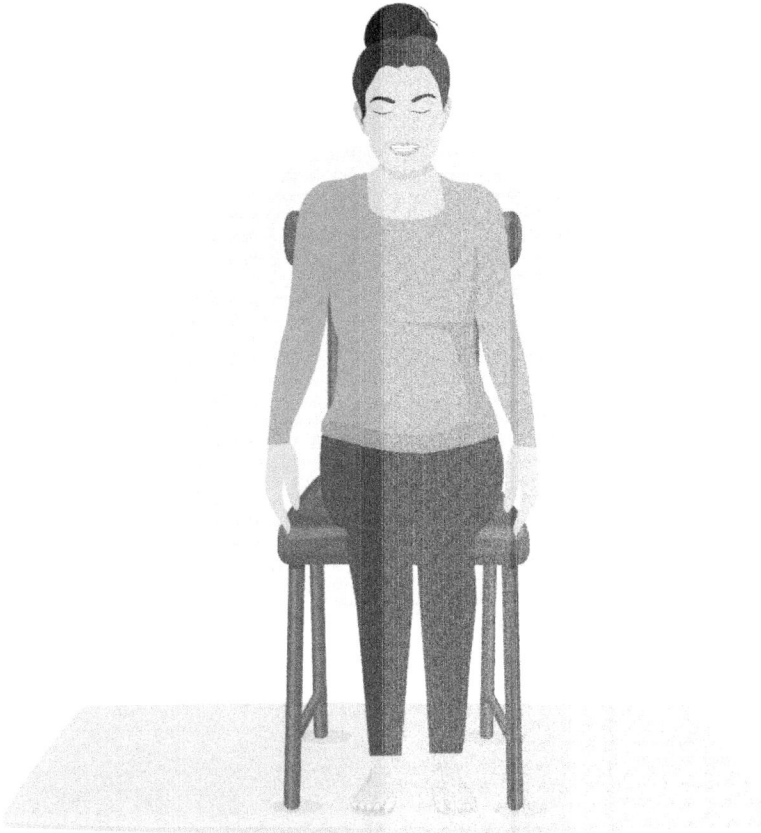

This exercise stretches your face: your lips and mouth in particular. It also helps boost happiness and keep you positive.

Step-by-Step Instructions

- Sit up tall and comfortable at the edge of the chair with your spine erect and relaxed, feet flat on the floor at about hip-width apart.

- Rest your hands on your upper thighs just above your knees and take a deep breath in through your nose and slowly exhale.

- Smile as wide as you can, stretching the entire mouth. Hold there for a few seconds

- Relax your lips and mouth

- Repeat.

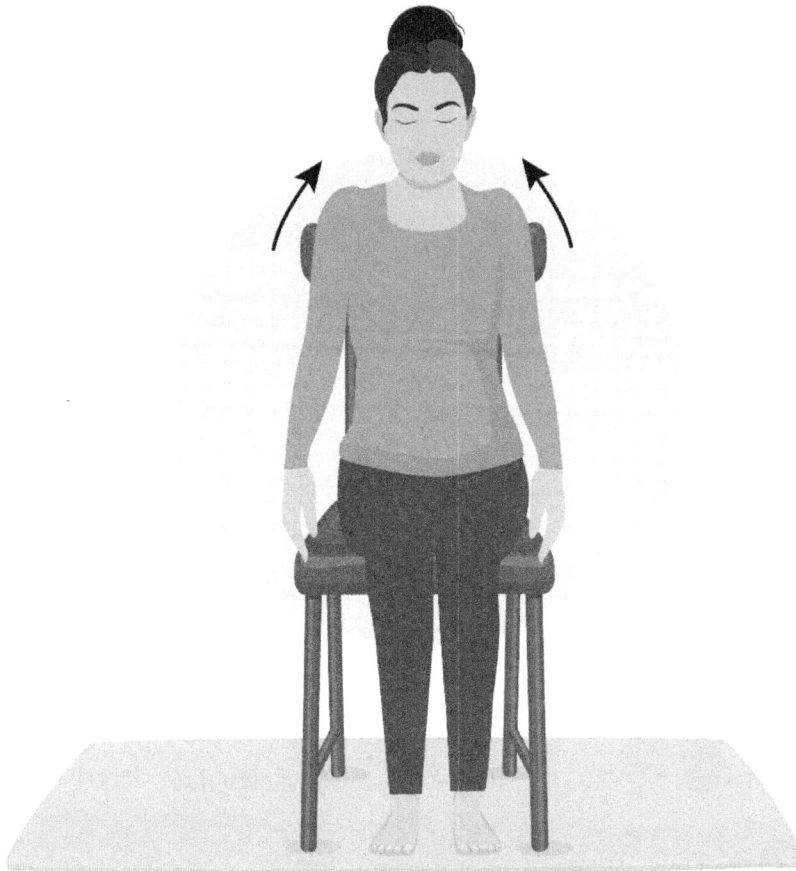

We tend to hold a lot of tension on our shoulders. Shoulder shrugs over exaggerate the tension then finally lets it go fully. You can try this exercise if you feel stressed and want to let go of the stress in your shoulders or if you want to quickly release the edginess in your shoulders, body, and mind. It also helps strengthen your shoulder muscles. This move works out your shoulders and lats.

Step-by-Step Instructions

- Sit upright in the chair so that your back isn't leaning on the chair

- Keep your feet flat and firmly planted on the floor at a hip distance apart with your palms on your thighs and shoulders relaxed.

- Take a deep breath in through your nose, lifting both shoulders towards your ears (as if you are cold).

- Hold the tensed position for about three seconds.

- Then, release the shoulders fully as you breathe out.

- Repeat.

Elbow Extensions

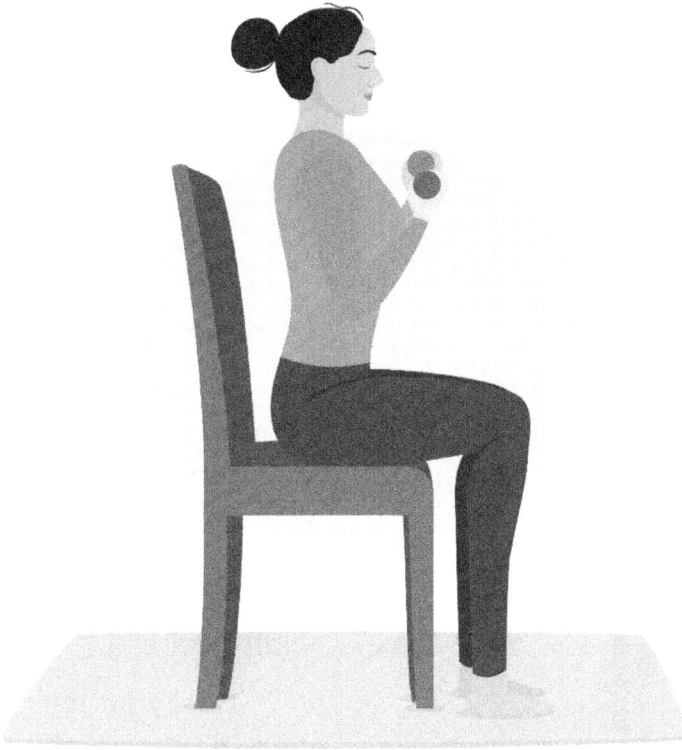

This exercise works out your arms and shoulders. It helps increase circulation in these areas, improve elbow joint mobility and strengthen the muscles in your upper arms and shoulders.

Step-by-Step Instructions

- Sit up tall and comfortable towards the edge of the chair with your spine erect and relaxed, feet flat on the floor at about hip-width apart.

- Rest your hands on your upper thighs just above your knees and take a deep breath in through your nose and slowly exhale.

- Extend your arms to your sides with your palms facing forward.

- Lift them as if you are curling your biceps and bring your fingertips to your shoulders

- Repeat.

Arm Circles

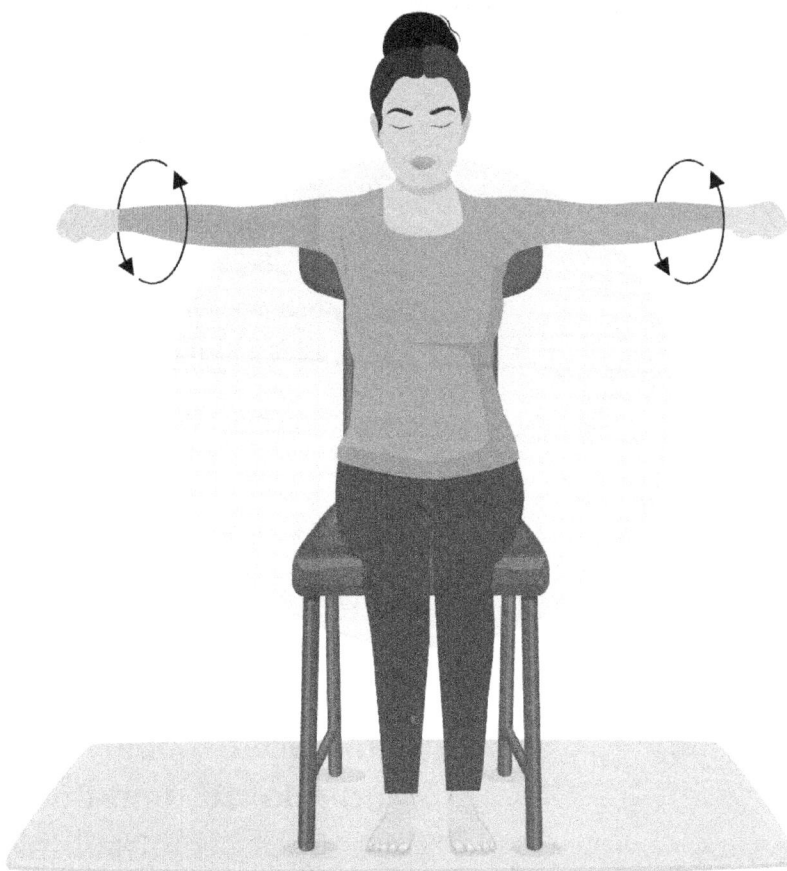

This exercise helps work out your arms and shoulders. It helps strengthen the muscles of your arms and improve shoulder joint flexibility.

Step-by-Step Instructions

- Sit up tall and comfortable towards the edge of the chair with your spine erect and relaxed, feet flat on the floor at about hip-width apart.

- Rest your hands on your upper thighs just above your knees and take a deep breath in through your nose and slowly exhale.

- Extend your arms straight out at your sides with your palms facing the floor.

- Slowly make small circles in a forward motion. Ensure that your shoulders are down and relaxed.

- Start increasing the size of the circles and without lowering your hands, switch the direction to backward motion starting with small circles as you make them bigger.

- After several breaths, lower your arms back to your sides and shake them gently.

- Repeat.

Hand pulls

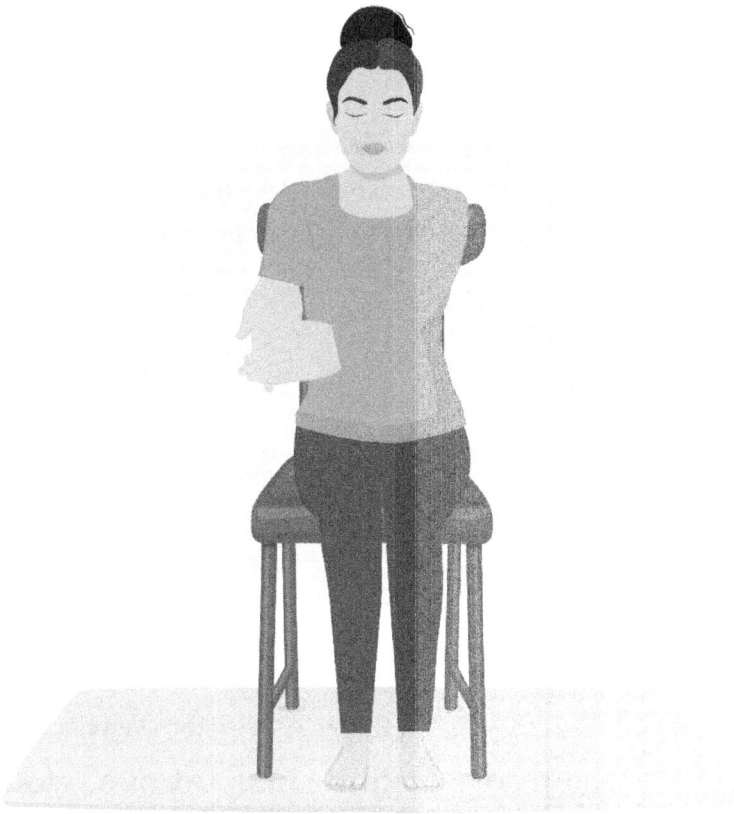

This exercise is one of the simplest stretches that tells you how tight your forearms, hands, and wrists are. Hand pulls work out your hands, wrists, and forearms. It helps relieve cramping and achiness in your fingers, forearms, and wrists. It also helps relieve anxiety and keeps your mind focused.

Step-by-Step Instructions

- Sit up tall and comfortable towards the edge of the chair with your spine erect and relaxed, feet flat on the floor at about hip-width apart, and a straight back.

- Rest your hands on your upper thighs just above your knees and take a deep breath in through your nose and slowly exhale.

- Extend your right arm straight out in front of you with palms facing down.

- Bring your left arm and pull the right-hand fingers back towards the torso. Hold there for a few breaths as you pull the fingers.

- Now, turn your right arm such that the palms face down, bring your left hand over it and press its back down. Hold for a few breaths.

- Lastly, turn the right palm up to face the ceiling and use your left hand to pull its fingers down holding for a few breaths.

- Repeat alternating the hands.

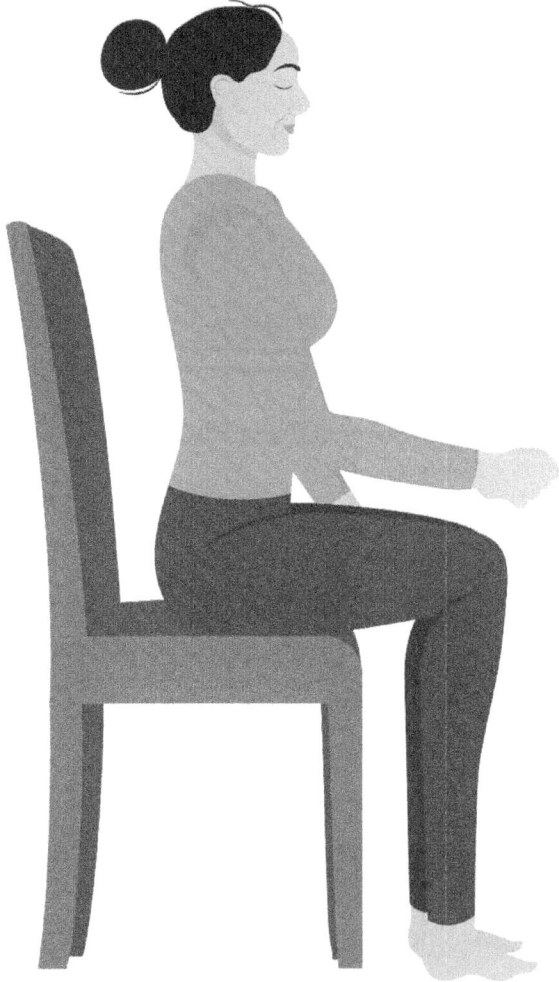

Wrist extensions work out your wrists, hands, and shoulders. They help strengthen your hand and shoulder muscles. This exercise also increases circulation in the hands and arms and helps improve the flexibility and mobility of wrist joints.

Step-by-Step Instructions

• Sit up tall and comfortable towards the edge of the chair with your spine erect and relaxed, feet flat on the floor at about hip-width apart, and a straight back.

• Rest your hands on your upper thighs just above your knees and take a deep breath in through your nose and slowly exhale.

• Extend both arms straight out in front of you.

• Extend your hands farther from the wrists so that your palms are facing away from you

• Flex your hands from the wrists to turn your palms so that they face your chest

• Repeat.

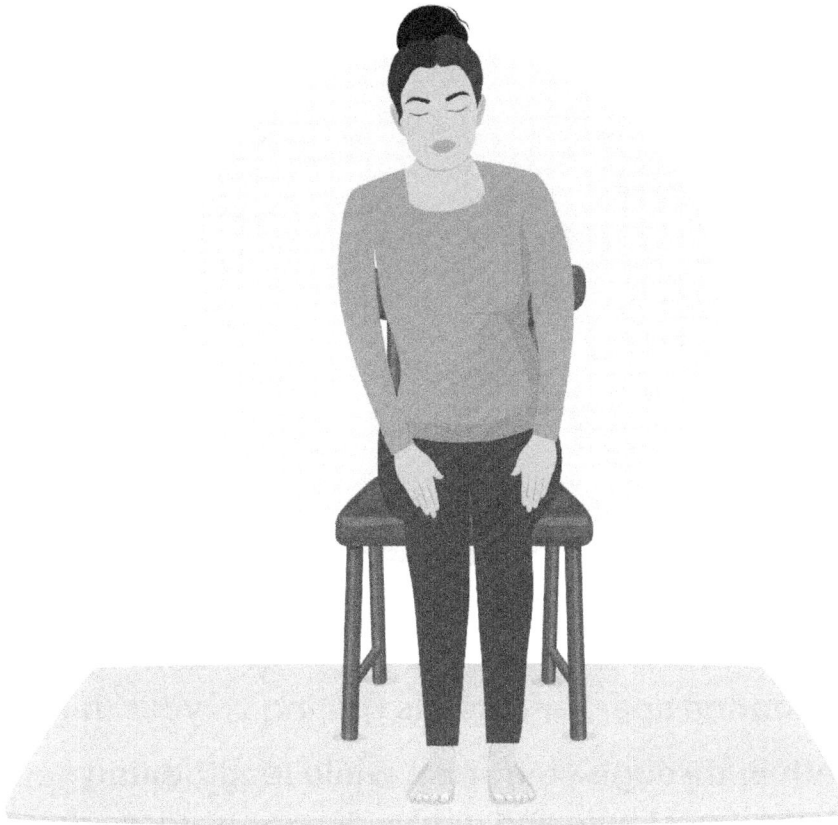

Side-to-Sides

This exercise works your obliques, core, waist, and lower back. It helps stretch and strengthen the muscles in these areas. You can also try this move if you want to keep creative juices flowing, or want to tone your midsection.

Step-by-Step Instructions

- Sit up tall and comfortable towards the edge of the chair with your spine erect and relaxed, feet flat on the floor at about hip-width apart, and a straight back.

- Rest your hands on your upper thighs just above your knees and take a deep breath in through your nose and slowly exhale.

- Breathe in as you slide your ribcage to the right. Don't move your legs and lower body.

- Breathe out as you slide the ribcage to the left in the same way.

- Repeat moving left and right at your desired pace.

Seated Forward Bend

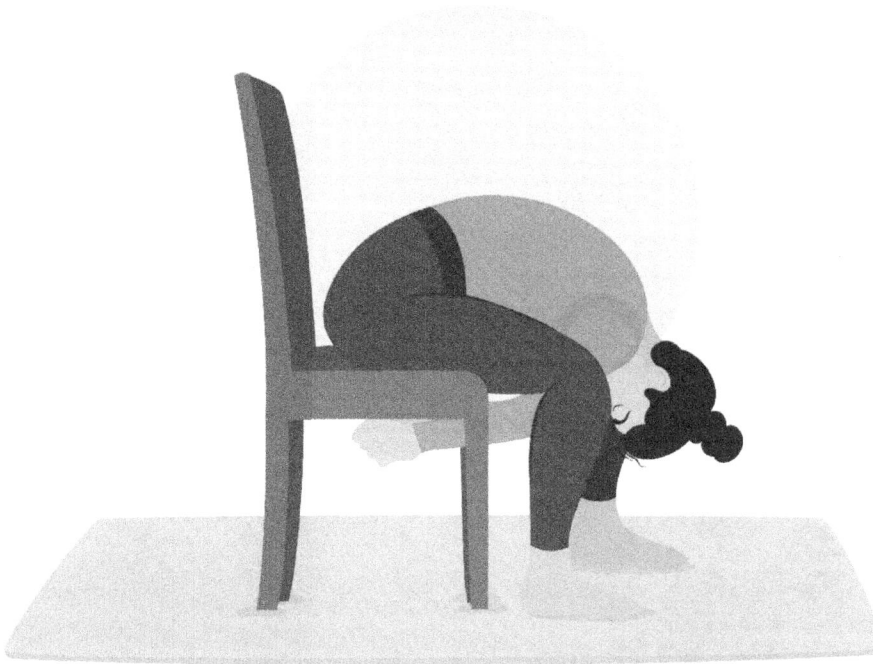

This exercise works out your back, hips, and legs. It helps gain flexibility and mobility in the hips and lower back. It also helps relieve anxiety, stress, and tension.

Step-by-Step Instructions

- Sit up tall in the chair, with your feet planted flat on the floor at a hip distance apart and palms resting on your thighs.

- Take a deep breath in through your nose while lengthening your spine, then exhale as you slowly and gently drop your torso down and let your belly rest on your thighs.

- Lower your hands and touch the floor on your palms.

- Keep your neck relaxed and release your head hanging down

- Hold there for 3-5 deep inhales and exhales

- Then, press your arms gently into the floor and lift your torso slowly to return to a seated position. If you can't reach down, just rest your head on your laps and wrap your hands behind your knees.

- Repeat.

Single Leg Stretch

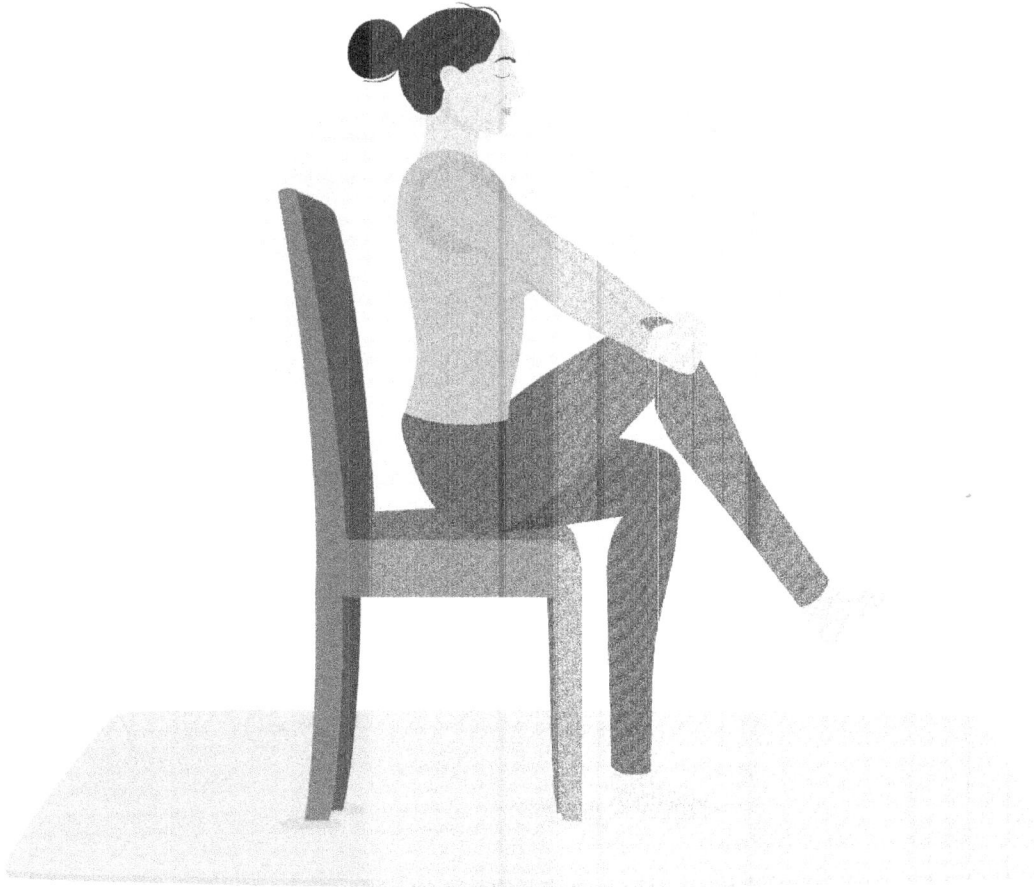

This exercise works out your hamstrings, hips, and lower back. It helps gain hamstring and hip flexibility and joint mobility. It also helps release tension from these muscles.

Step-by-Step Instructions

- Sit up tall and comfortable towards the edge of the chair with your spine erect and relaxed, feet planted firmly on the floor at about hip-width apart.

- Rest your hands on your upper thighs just above your knees and take a deep breath in through your nose and slowly exhale.

- Extend one leg in front of you with the heel touching the floor and the foot flexed.

- Breathe in and lengthen your spine, then exhale slowly as you gently bend your torso forward.

- Place your hands on the thigh of the extended leg.

- Take a gaze at the toes of the extended leg and keep bending forward to lengthen your spine as much as you can.

- Hold there for 3-5 deep breaths.

- Return to the upright sitting position by pressing into your hands gently to lift your spine back upright.

- Repeat on the opposite side.

Warrior I (Virabhadrasana I)

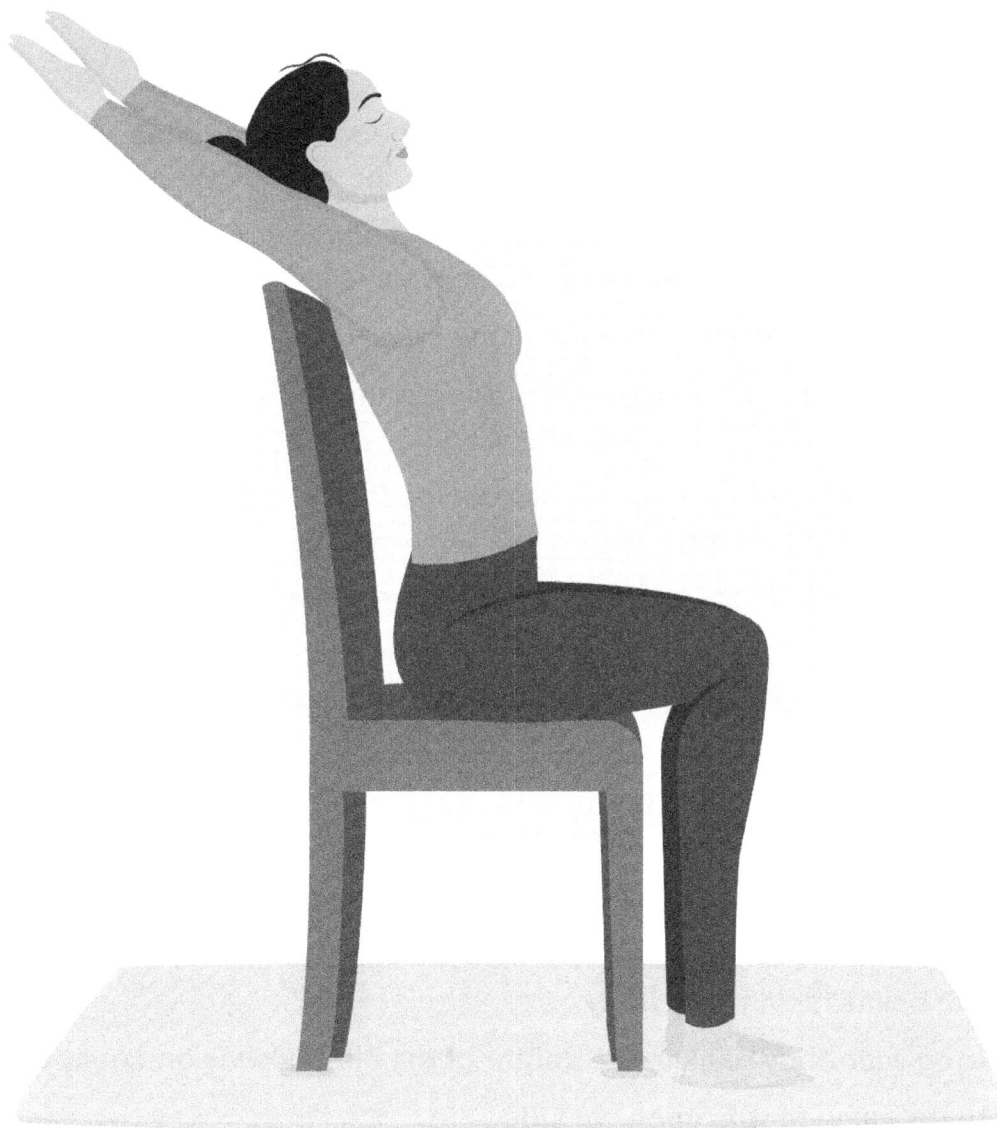

This pose helps strengthen and stretch your outer hips, buttocks, quadriceps, hamstrings, and inner thighs. Always try warrior 1 whenever you feel shaky or unsteady, need some confidence, or want to boost the strength of your lower half in general.

Step-by-Step Instructions

- Sit up tall and comfortable towards the edge of the chair with your spine erect and relaxed, feet planted firmly on the floor at about hip-width apart.

- Rest your hands on your upper thighs just above your knees and take a deep breath in through your nose and slowly exhale.

- Reach around to hold the back of the chair for support.

- Keep the right hip on the chair, and extend the left leg towards the floor, aligning the knee below the left hip.

- Gently tug that hip and press through the foot until you feel the stretch along the front of your thigh.

- To deepen the pose, simply walk away farther back.

- Now raise your arms and stretch up to lengthen the front of your body, or place the hands above your head with palms together and gaze at them.

- If you struggle with flexibility or mobility, you can just keep your palms facing each other in front of you at a shoulder distance apart instead of raising your hands above your head.

- Feel confident in your pose and hold it for 3-5 deep inhales and exhales.

- On your final exhale, gently and slowly bring your hands down by your sides with palms facing your body.

- Bring your body back to the center of the chair slowly and gently.

- Do the same for the opposite side.

- Repeat alternating the sides.

Chair Downward Facing Dog (Adho Mukha Svanasana)

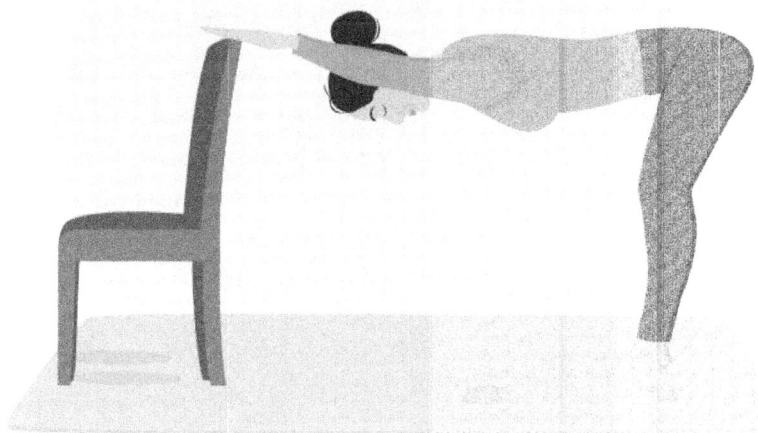

This pose works out your arms, back, hips and legs. It is very helpful if you want to improve your balance, gain flexibility in the back muscles, and strengthen your legs.

Step-by-Step Instructions

- Stand up tall in front of the chair facing it. Your feet should be parallel to each other at hip-width apart.

- Take a deep breath in and out then hold the chair seat with both hands. Ensure that you feel stable and relaxed.

- Make a few steps backward until you feel your spine is properly straightened.

- Hold there for 5-10 deep breaths

- Slowly return to the standing position by gently walking your feet back towards the chair while still holding onto the chair seat for support.

- Repeat.

Leg lifts

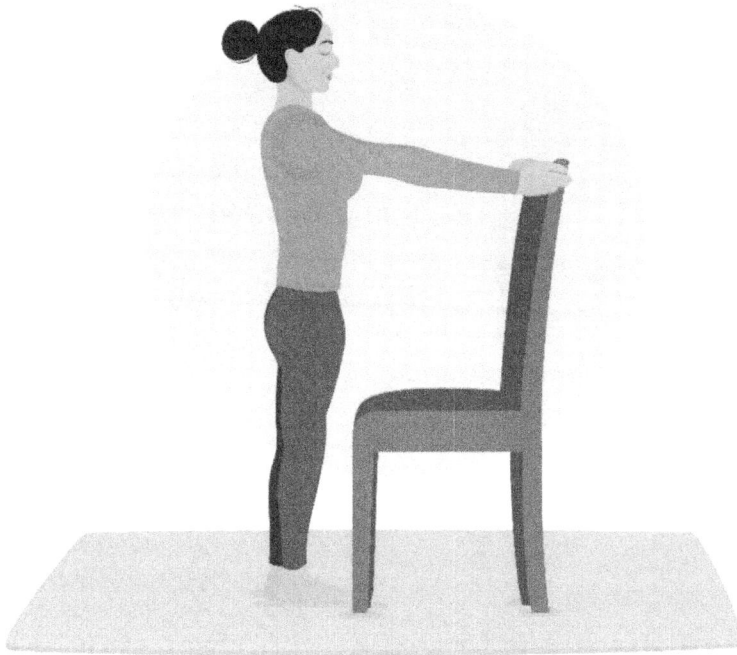

This exercise works your core, hip flexors, psoas, pelvic floor muscles, and inner thighs. It helps tone and strengthen your abdominals. It also helps relieve restlessness and leg cramps and helps boost your energy and focus.

Step-by-Step Instructions

- Sit up tall and comfortable towards the edge of the chair with your spine erect and relaxed, feet flat on the floor at about hip-width apart, and a straight back.

- Rest your hands on your upper thighs just above your knees and take a deep breath in through your nose and slowly exhale.

- Bring your hands and hold the edges of your chair seat

- Engage your abdominals and focus on lifting your right leg a few inches off the ground. Hold there for a few seconds then lower it back and lift the left leg the same way.

- Repeat alternating the legs.

Seated Knee Hugs

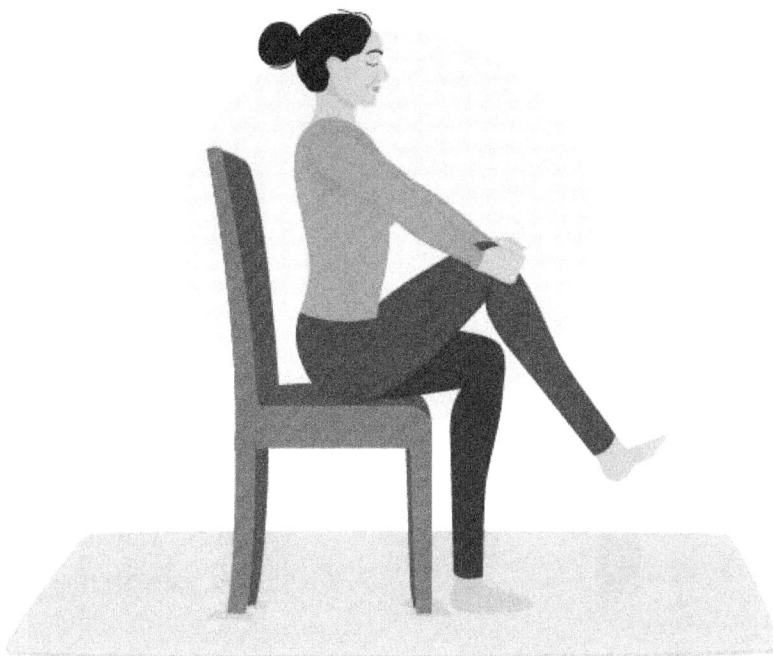

This pose helps strengthen the muscles surrounding your shoulders, legs, and hips. It also improves the mobility and flexibility of the knee and hip joints.

Step-by-Step Instructions

- **Sit up tall and comfortable towards the edge of the chair with** your spine erect and relaxed, feet planted firmly on the floor at about hip-width apart.

- Rest your hands on your upper thighs just above your knees and take a deep breath in through your nose and slowly exhale.

- Slowly pull your right knee towards your chest.

- Hold there for about 3-5 relaxed breaths.

- Slowly lower the leg down to the floor.

- Repeat for the opposite leg.

Seated Heel Raises

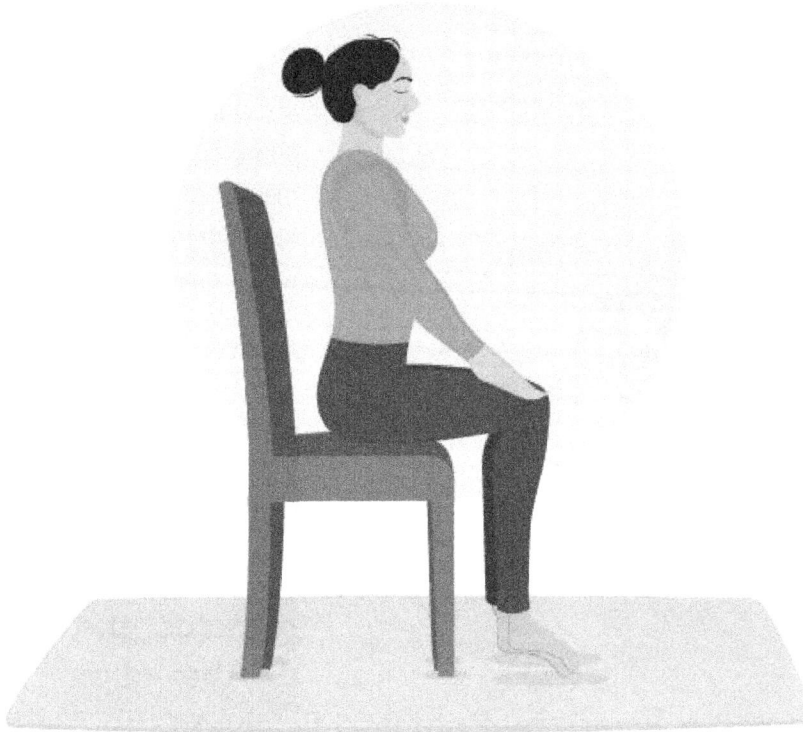

This pose engages the calf muscles and inner thighs. Heel raises help work out the opposite sides of your feet and the lower legs. They improve mobility and flexibility of the ankle joint and boost our moods. Try this pose when you need positive energy, want to strengthen your calves, or need to relieve stress and anxiety.

Step-by-Step Instructions

- Sit up tall and comfortable towards the edge of the chair with your spine erect and relaxed.

- Rest your hands on your upper thighs just above your knees and take a deep breath in through your nose and slowly exhale.

- Inhale as you lift both heels then exhale as you lower them.

- Repeat.

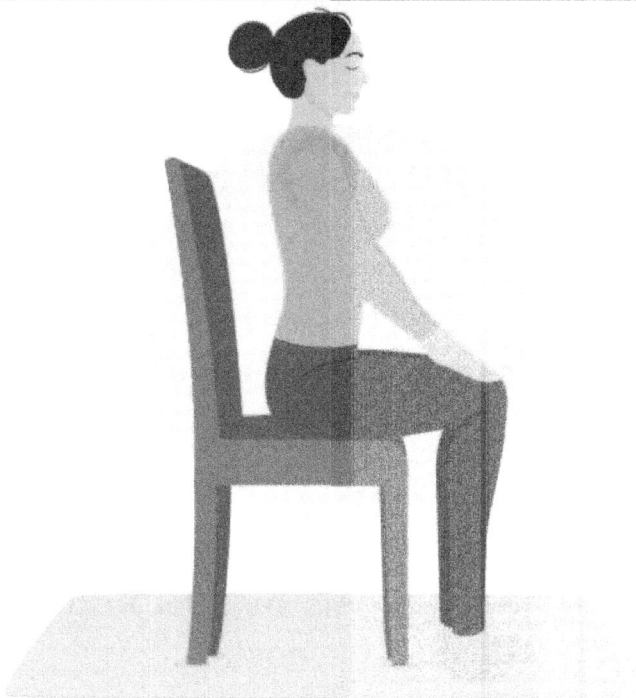

This pose helps stretch and strengthen your toes and feet. It is also helpful in improving foot stability and mobility.

Step-by-Step Instructions

- Sit up tall and comfortable towards the edge of the chair with your spine erect and relaxed, feet flat on the floor at about hip-width apart.

- Rest your hands on your upper thighs just above your knees and take a deep breath in through your nose and slowly exhale.

- Keeping the ball of your feet firmly planted on the floor, lift your toes up and curl them under.

- Hold there for about 3-5 deep breaths.

- Repeat.

Standing Chair Warrior I

This pose helps stretch and strengthen your abdominals, arms, and leg muscles.

Step-by-Step Instructions

- Stand next to your chair: either behind it or by the side and rest your right hand on the chair back.

- Make a full leg length step backward with your left foot and tilt it so that it is angled at about 75 degrees forward.

- Bend your right knee until the thigh gets parallel to the floor. Ensure that your knee doesn't go past the ankle.

- Lift your left arm above your ears. For a challenging pose, lift both arms above your ears with palms facing each other and completely press them against each other.

- Hold here for about 3 to 5 breaths and repeat on the other side.

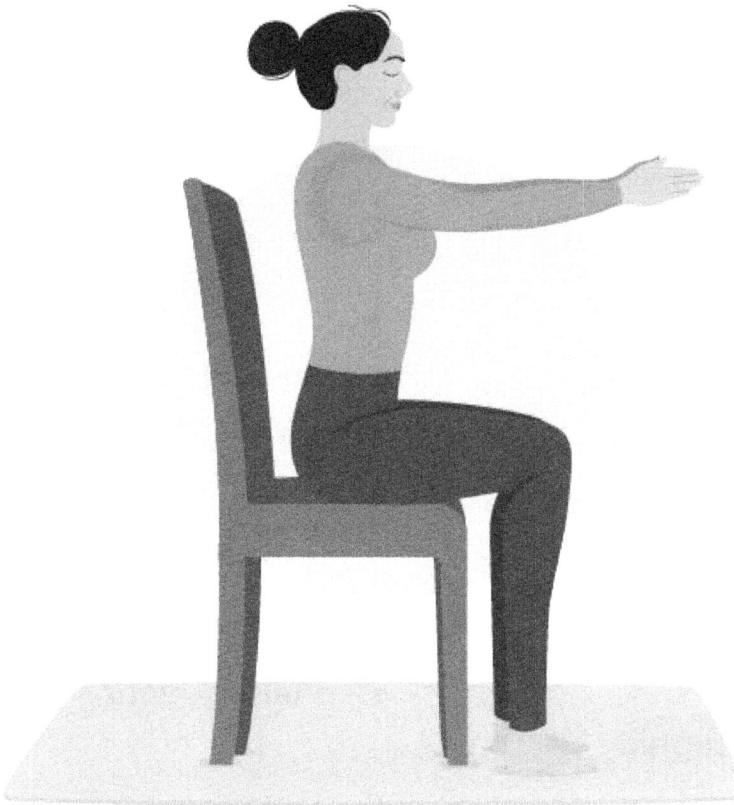

Palming

This pose will help you calm down and feel good after your yoga exercises.

Step-by-Step Instructions

- Sit tall and comfortable in your chair

- Bring your palms together and rub them against each other until you feel warmth in them

- Cup them slightly and gently place them over your face covering your eyes. You may close your eyes or keep them open.

- Feel the warmth of the palms on your eyes. Ensure not to put pressure on your eyeballs.

- Hold the pose for about three to five minutes.

Cooling Breath (Sithali)

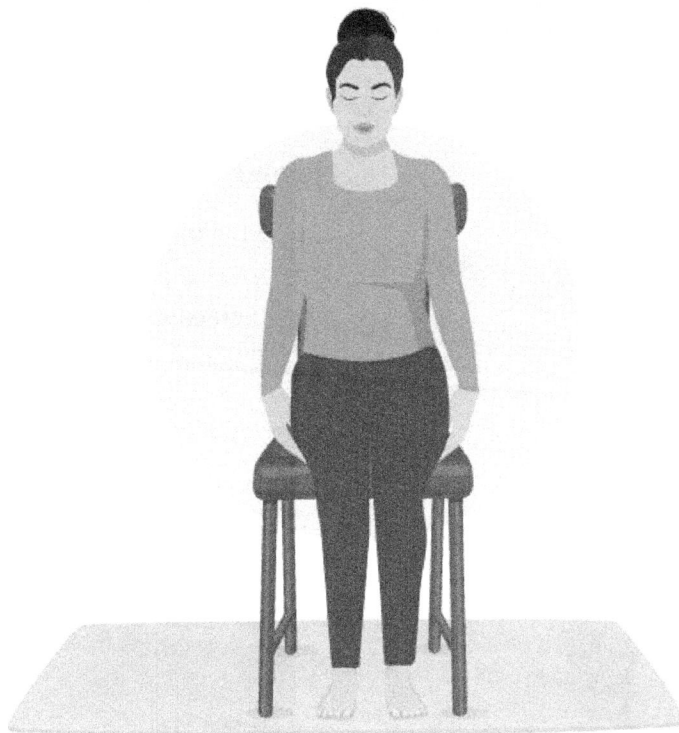

As mentioned earlier, Sithali will help you cool down and calm your body after performing your yoga sessions.

Step-by-Step Instructions

• Sit up tall in the chair with your hips towards the edge of the chair, back straight, your feet planted firmly on the floor at a hip-width apart.

• Place your palms face-down on your thighs.

• Take deep breaths in and out twice or thrice through your nose to prepare for this pranayama.

• Curl the sides of your tongue inwards towards the center to roll it into a tube-like shape. If you can't roll your tongue, purse your lips to make a small "o" shape with your mouth.

• Inhale slowly through the tube if you roll your tongue or channel the air through the "o" shaped opening if your lips are pursed.

• Close your mouth and breathe out slowly through your nose.

• Repeat until you feel the maximum cooling effect.

Final Relaxation and Meditation

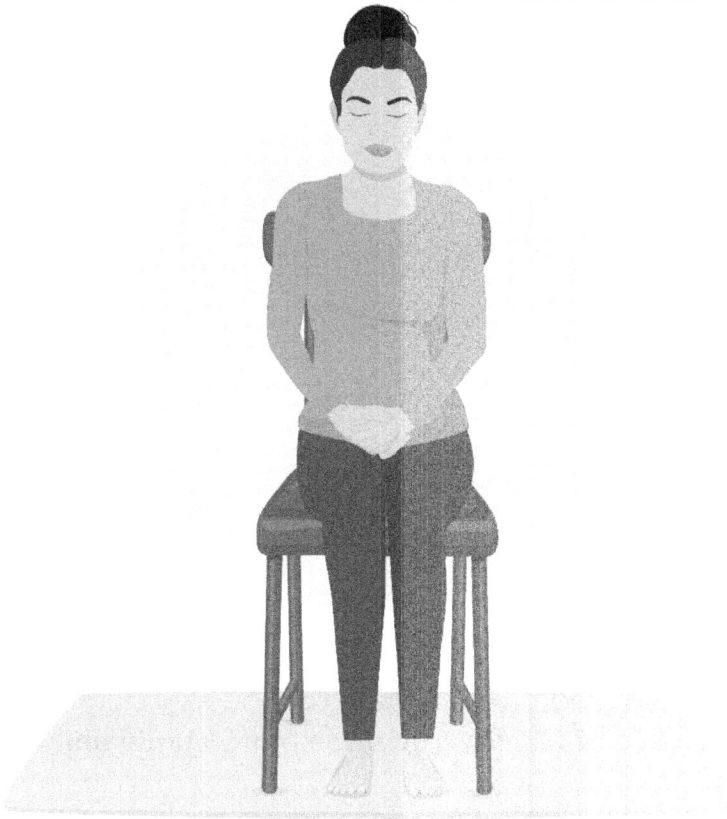

After your yoga exercises, it is very important to relax your body. The final relaxation pose makes you feel good, calms, and gives your body time to start integrating the results of your yoga practice.

Step-by-Step Instructions

- Sit up tall and comfortable at the edge of the chair with your spine erect and relaxed, feet flat on the floor at about hip-width apart. Raise your feet using a bolster or a folded blanket if they can't touch the ground when seated.

- Rest your hands on your upper thighs just above your knees and feel the weight of your body on the seat. Sense the chair as if it is your first time sitting on it. Try to move gently from side to side in the chair and notice how your hips feel in the chair and how your feet feel on the ground.

- Relax your shoulders and hands and allow your breath to flow naturally. With your eyes closed, become aware of your breath. Pay attention to it as you inhale and exhale through your nose. Ensure not to change your breath. Just pay attention to it. Notice if it is strained or relaxed, its length and temperature as it comes in and out of your body.

- Come back from the meditation after one or two minutes.

You are done!

Enjoy the rest of your day!

Please try to do this routine three to five times every week and stay consistent. It is through being consistent that you will reap the most out of its benefits.

After a few weeks, you will be ready for intermediate routine exercises in the next chapter which are a bit intense and require you to be more stable and a bit flexible.

Chapter Four:
Our Dedicated Intermediate Program

In this chapter, you will find our dedicated intermediate program. The chair yoga exercises in this program are more dynamic and tailored to the intermediate level. Once you are done with the routine in the first chapter, you are ready for this chapter's routine. If you are not new to chair yoga, this sequence of exercises can help you enhance your chair yoga practice. You can also use these exercises to add some more challenging elements to your yoga practice.

You can perform these exercises as a stand-alone routine or in a combination with the warm-up sequence from chapter two. But is it important to prepare our mind and breathing system in order to increase our concentration level during the exercise. So we will start with a breathing exercise. **Let's get into the routine!**

Cleansing Breath (Kapalbhati)

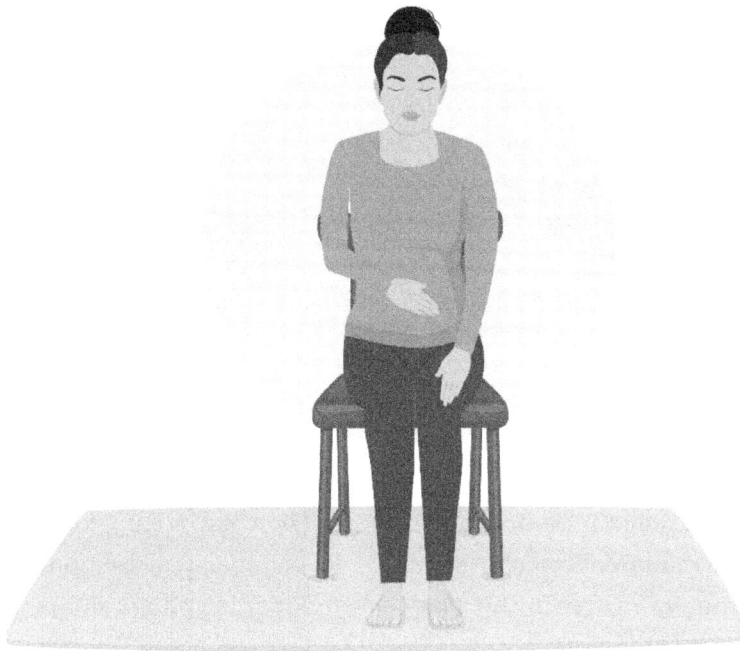

- Sit up tall in the chair leaving some space behind you so that you are not leaning on it.

- Plant your feet flat and firmly on the floor with your hands hanging by your sides

- Keep your left hand relaxed by your side and put your right hand on your belly

- Take a deep full breath in through your nose, then breathe out all the air as you pull your navel and the belly back towards the spine. Next, take a partial breath in and exhale quickly through the nose relaxing the navel and the abdomen. You may pump at a pace of your choice. Just ensure that the breath is continuous but the "breathe-ins" are very subtle and small. Perform as many pumps as you can. Start smaller and build your way up.

- On the last pump, stop and take a full breath in and a full breath out.

Seated Head Tilt

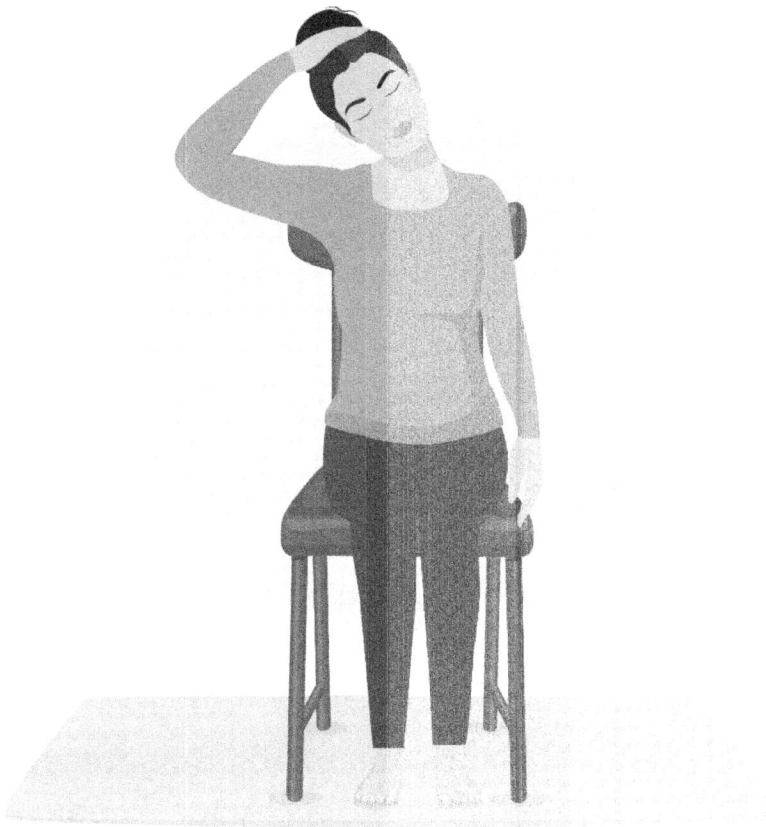

Head tilts workout and stretches the muscles surrounding your neck. They help improve flexibility and mobility of the neck.

Step-by-Step Instructions

- Sit up tall and comfortable at the edge of the chair with your spine erect and relaxed, feet flat on the floor at about hip-width apart.

- Rest your hands on your upper thighs just above your knees and take a deep breath in through your nose and slowly exhale.

- Tip your head gently to the left, then bring it back to the center.

- Tip it to the right, then bring it to the center again.

- Repeat.

Close/Open (Eye Movement)

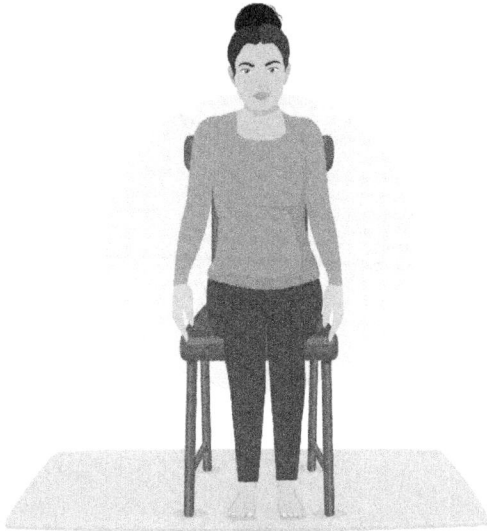

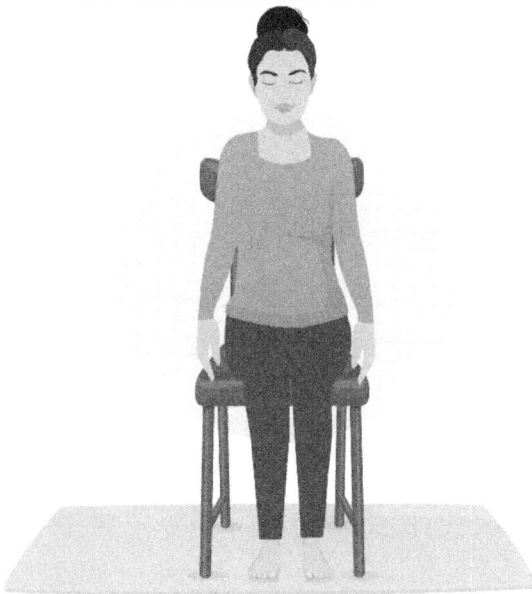

This movement helps us notice the difference between using our external environment and our internal feelings for information. Closing your eyes is the best way to scan yourself internally. Try making this movement when you feel that your eyes are tired or need to boost your mindset.

Step-by-Step Instructions

- Sit up tall and comfortable at the edge of the chair with your spine erect and relaxed, feet flat on the floor at about hip-width apart.

- Rest your hands on your upper thighs just above your knees and take a deep breath in through your nose and slowly exhale.

- Close your eyes as you inhale deeply, then exhale as you open them as wide as you can

- Repeat.

Open wide (Mouth movement)

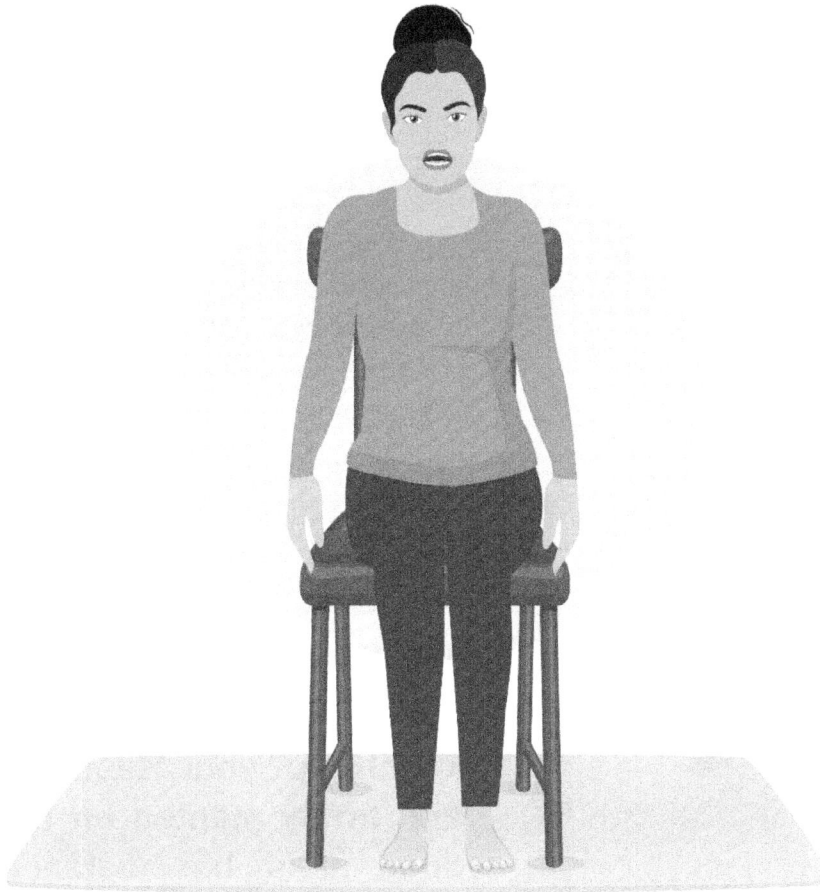

This exercise helps release tension from your entire body and mind letting everything go. It helps stretch your entire face muscles too.

Step-by-Step Instructions

- Sit up tall and comfortable at the edge of the chair with your spine erect and relaxed, feet flat on the floor at about hip-width apart.

- Rest your hands on your upper thighs just above your knees and take a deep breath in through your nose and slowly exhale.

- Open your mouth as wide as you can. Hold there for a few seconds

- Relax your lips and mouth to release the pose.

- Repeat.

Shoulder Rotations

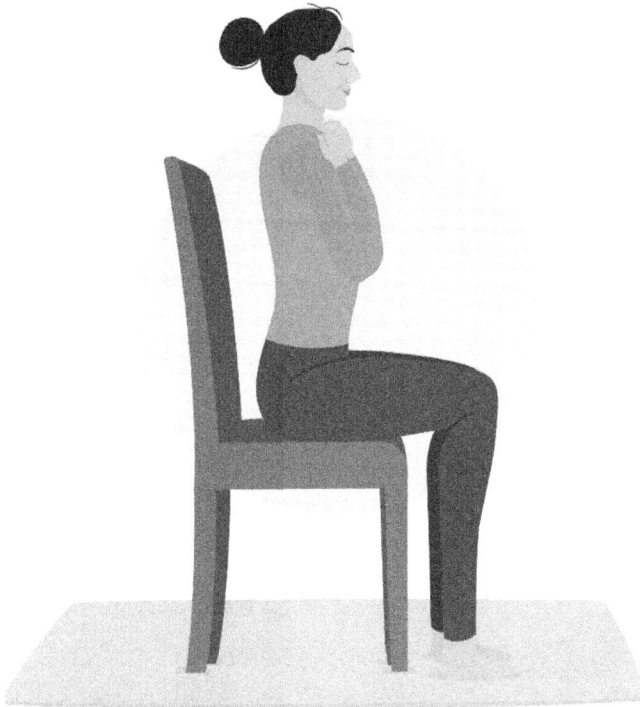

This exercise helps strengthen your upper arm and shoulder muscles. It also increases circulation in your shoulders and improves shoulder joint mobility.

Step-by-Step Instructions

- Sit upright in the chair so that your back isn't leaning on the chair

- Keep your feet flat and firmly planted on the floor at a hip distance apart with your palms on your thighs and shoulders relaxed.

- Bring both hands on your shoulders and hold your shoulder joints with your fingertips.

- Make circles with your elbows starting with moving in a clockwise direction and then anticlockwise.

- Repeat alternating the direction.

High Altar Arms

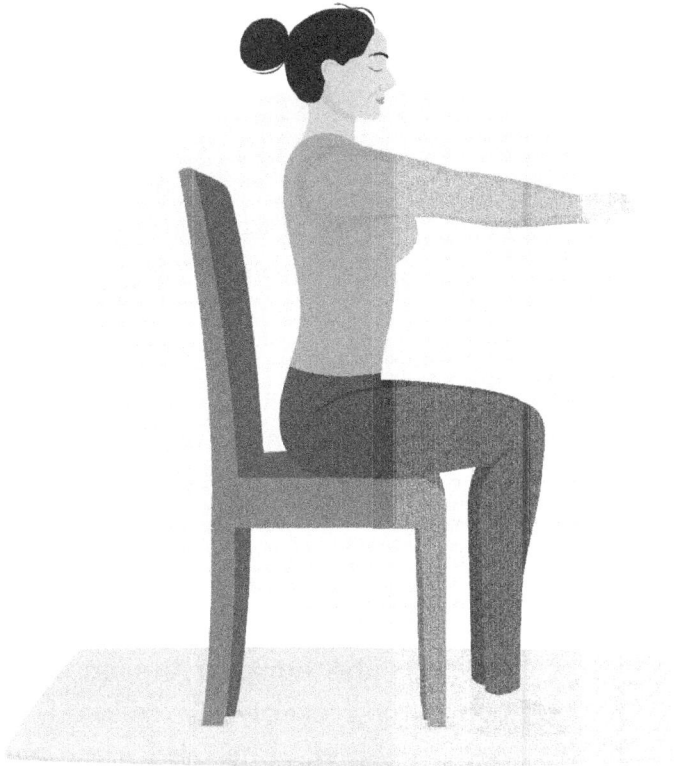

This move works your arms, wrists, shoulders, and the sides of your torso. It helps relieve your arms, shoulders, and wrists from tension. It also helps strengthen the muscles in these areas and give you positive energy.

Step-by-Step Instructions

- Sit up tall and comfortable towards the edge of the chair with your spine erect and relaxed, feet flat on the floor at about hip-width apart, and a straight back.

- Rest your hands on your upper thighs just above your knees and take a deep breath in through your nose and slowly exhale.

- Extend your arms straight out in front of you, interlace the fingers and keep the palms inverted such that they face away from your torso. Hold here for a few seconds and just feel the stretch.

- Keeping your ribs relaxed, raise your arms up above your head. Ensure that your shoulder tops remain down and stretch from elbow to wrist. Try to imagine that there is something on the altar created above you that you wish to bring into your life.

- Hold here for about 5-10 breaths then release your arms.

- Repeat.

Finger Extensions

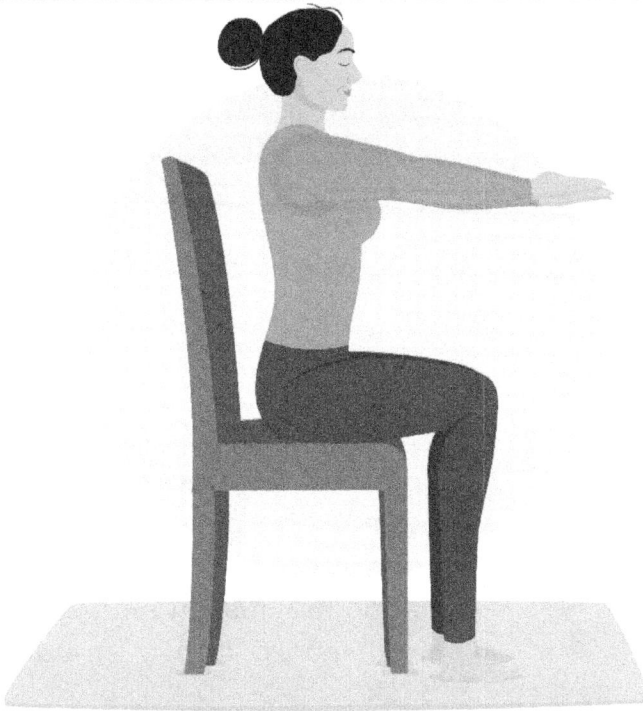

This exercise works out your finger joints, hands, arms, and shoulders. It stretches your fingers and helps strengthen your hand, arms, and shoulder muscles. It also increases circulation in the hands and arms and helps improve flexibility and mobility of your finger joints.

Step-by-Step Instructions

- Sit up tall and comfortable towards the edge of the chair with your spine erect and relaxed, feet flat on the floor at about hip-width apart, and a straight back.

- Rest your hands on your upper thighs just above your knees and take a deep breath in through your nose and slowly exhale.

- Extend both arms in front of you.

- Spread your fingers wide and hold for a few seconds.

- Then, close your fist into a ball and hold for a few seconds too.

- Repeat alternating between spreading the fingers and closing them into a fistball.

Wrist Rotations

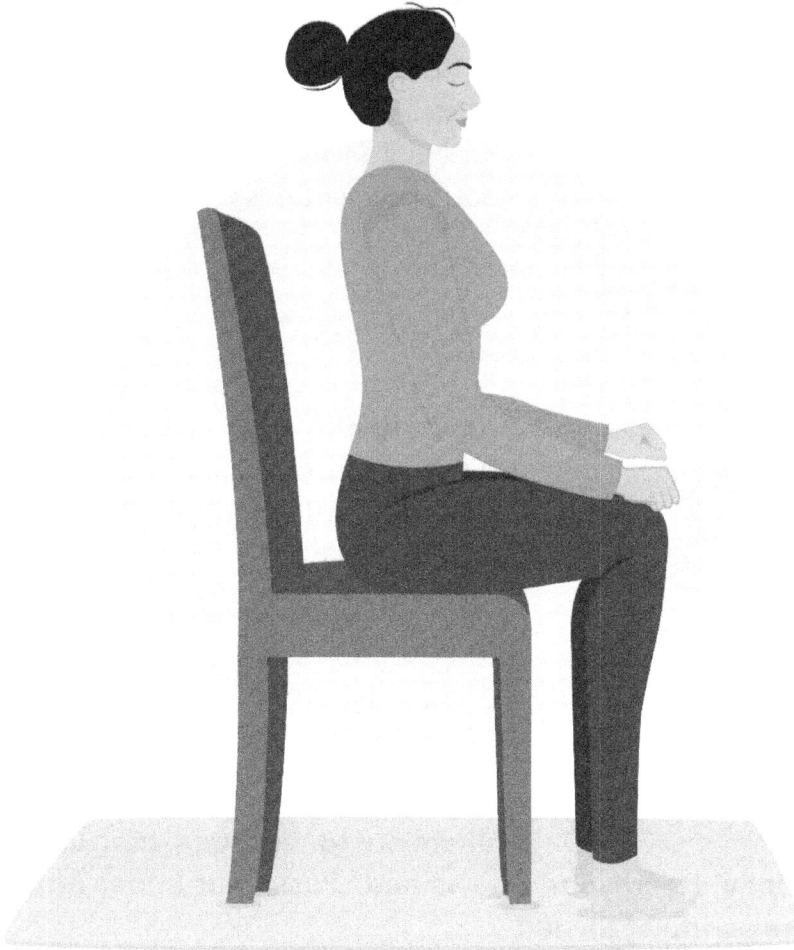

Wrist rotations work out your wrists, hands, and shoulders. They help strengthen your hand and shoulder muscles. This exercise also increases circulation in the hands and arms and helps improve the flexibility and mobility of wrist joints.

Step-by-Step Instructions

- **Sit up tall and comfortable towards the edge of the chair with your spine erect and relaxed, feet flat on the floor at about hip-width apart, and a straight back.**

- **Rest your hands on your upper thighs just above your knees and take a deep breath in through your nose and slowly exhale.**

- **Extend both arms straight out in front of you.**

- **Rotate your wrists in a clockwise direction, then rotate them in an anticlockwise direction.**

- **Repeat.**

Eagle Arms (Chair Garudasana)

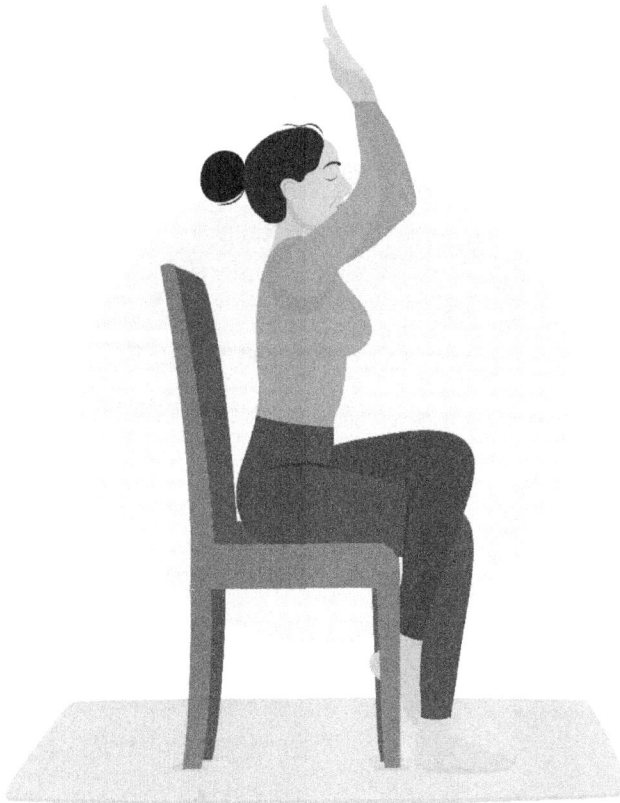

This posture works out your arms, upper back, and shoulders. It is perfect for stretching and gaining flexibility and mobility in these muscles. It also helps increase your focus and concentration.

Step-by-Step Instructions

• Sit up tall and comfortable towards the edge of the chair with your spine erect and relaxed, feet planted firmly on the floor at about hip-width apart.

• Rest your hands on your upper thighs just above your knees and take a deep breath in through your nose and slowly exhale.

• Now drop your hands to reach them out to the sides, then lift them to the front of your body. Bend your elbows and cross your upper arms by bringing the right one on top of the left.

• Bring your right leg on top of your left thigh such that they are crossed.

• Keep your forearms wrapped around each other and bring your palms so they meet in front of your face. Your upper arms should be parallel to your thighs.

• Hold this position for 5-10 deep breaths

• Unwrap your arms and legs to release yourself from the cross position and return to sitting upright.

• Repeat for the opposite side.

Extended Side Angle

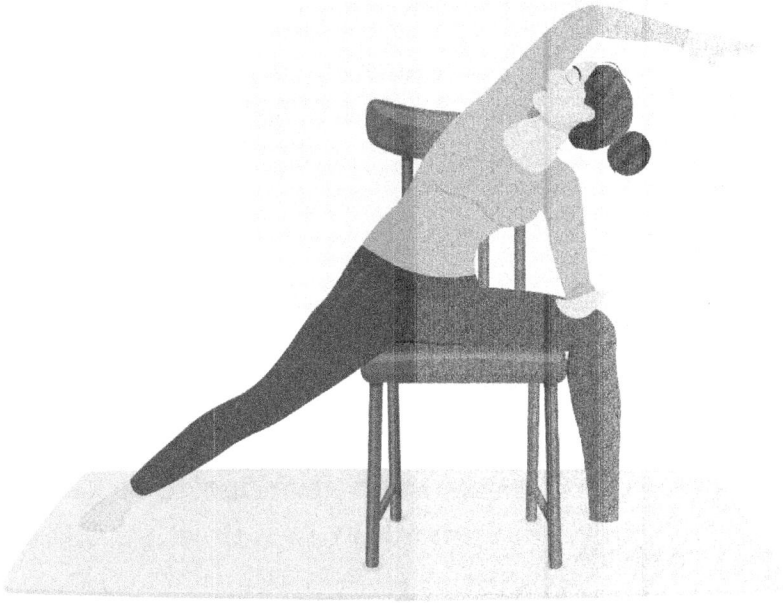

This is an amazing stretch, but it requires more space around you. This exercise works your hips, legs, and lower back. It helps stretch and strengthen the muscles of the hips, legs, and lower back. It also improves flexibility and mobility of the hip joint and increases the flow of oxygen to the lungs.

Step-by-Step Instructions

- Sit up tall and comfortable towards the edge of the chair with your spine erect and relaxed, feet flat on the floor at about hip-width apart, and a straight back.

- Rest your hands on your upper thighs just above your knees and take a deep breath in through your nose and slowly exhale.

- Open your right knee turning the right foot out at 90 degrees to the side

- Straighten your left leg and angle its foot in about 75 degrees as if you are coming into a seated warrior II position.

- From this position, rest your right forearm on your right knee with your palm facing upward.

- Using the back of the arm, push the knee more to the right.

- Feel the stretch and reach from the outer left foot all the way through the left fingers.

- Hold there for about 5-10 breaths.

- Slowly and gently release the pose and do the same to the opposite side.

- Repeat alternating the sides.

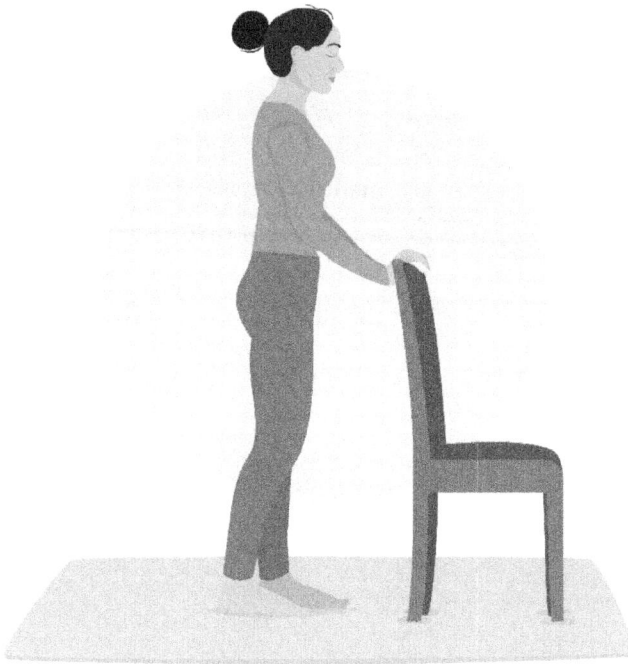

This stretch works out your hips, hands, torso, back, and thigh muscles. It helps improve flexibility and mobility of the hip joint.

Step-by-Step Instruction

- Stand up tall behind a chair facing its back about a foot away from it. Your feet should be parallel to each other at hip-width apart.

- Take a deep breath in and out then hold the back of the chair with both hands. Ensure that you feel stable and relaxed.

- Keeping your knees over your ankles, and hips on your knees, slowly bend forward from your hips. Hold here for about 3-5 deep breaths.

- For a deeper stretch, turn the chair so that the seat of the chair is facing you then hold the chair seat and bend forward from your hips. Ensure that your neck and back remain straight.

- Hold here for 3-5 deep breaths

- Repeat.

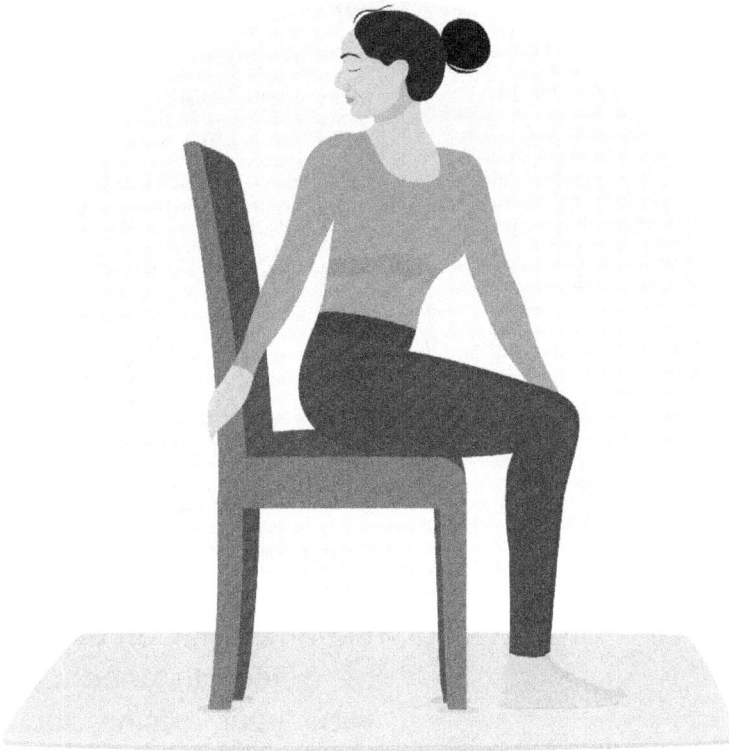

Seated Twist

This pose engages the back, neck, arms, and hips. It is helpful in gaining flexibility and joint mobility in the surrounding muscles. It also helps relieve tension and stiffness that may be caused by stress, trauma, and injury. Thanks to its twisting motion.

Step-by-Step Instructions

- Sit up tall in the chair leaving some space behind you. Plant your feet flat and firmly on the floor at a hip distance apart with your palms facing down on the upper side of your thighs.

- Take a deep breath in and out then place your left hand on your right thigh and the right hand on the chair seat behind you

- Breathe in as you lengthen your spine, then breathe out and twist your upper body towards the right. Look behind and go as far as you can.

- Hold there for 3-5 deep breaths.

- Unwind from the twist slowly and gently, returning to the center and uncrossing your leg, putting it back on the floor.

- Repeat for the opposite side.

Chair Pigeon Pose

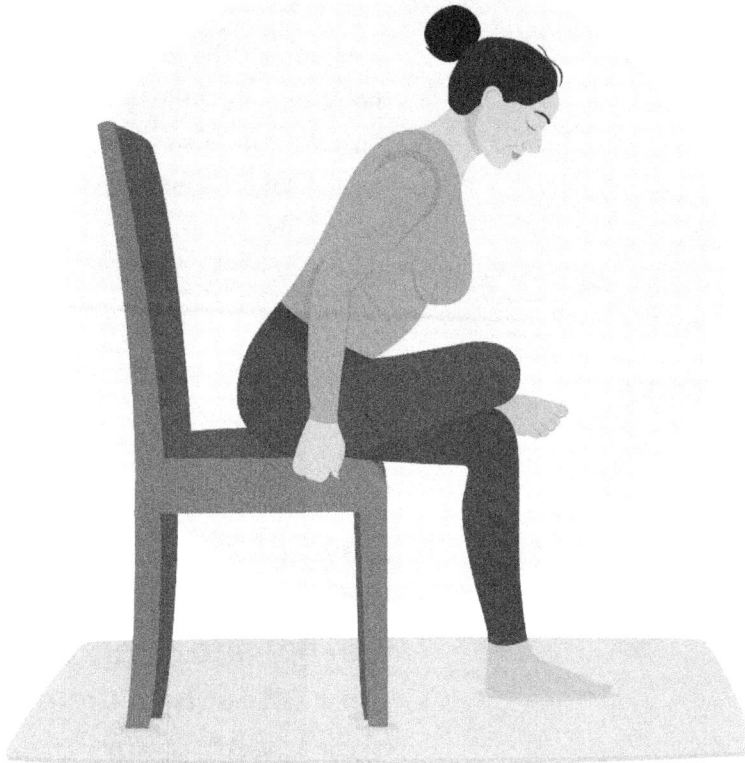

This exercise helps work out and strengthen your hamstrings, hips, lower back, glutes and thighs. Try it if you want to gain flexibility and mobility of your lower half and alleviate pain from sciatica or sciatic nerve irritation.

Step-by-Step Instructions

- Sit up tall in the chair leaving some space behind you. Plant your feet flat and firmly on the floor at a hip distance apart with your palms facing down on the upper side of your thighs.

- Take a deep breath in and out then bend your right leg and cross it over your left thigh at the right ankle keeping the right knee out to the side.

- For an easier variation, just bring your entire right leg and cross it on top of your left thigh.

- Rest your right hand on your shin and the left one on your right ankle, then tilt your torso forward slowly and gently maintaining a straight spine.

- Hold that posing for 3-5 deep inhales and exhales

- Next, slowly unwind from the position and bring your torso back to sitting upright.

- Repeat for the opposite leg.

Knee to Chest Pose (Eka Pada Apanasana)

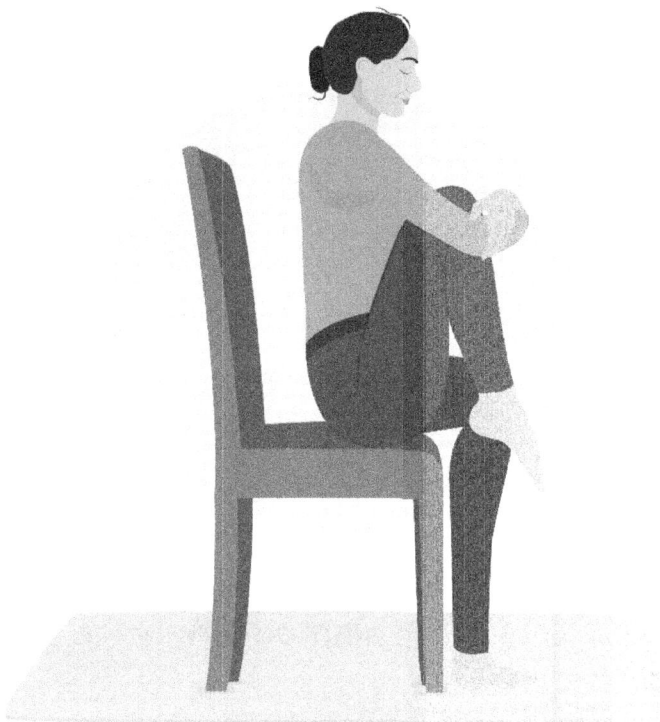

This pose works your abdominals, hips, and hamstrings. It is helpful in gaining flexibility in the hip and hamstring muscles. It also helps strengthen your abdominals gently.

Step-by-Step Instructions

- Sit up tall and comfortable towards the edge of the chair with your spine erect and relaxed, feet planted firmly on the floor at about hip-width apart.

- Rest your hands on your upper thighs just above your knees and take a deep breath in through your nose and slowly exhale.

- Raise your right leg towards your chest by bending the knee and holding it at the shin with both hands. The left leg should remain firmly planted on the floor.

- Now, flex your right foot

- Hold this position for 3-5 deep breaths

- Get back to the starting position by gently releasing your foot back to the floor

- Do the same for the opposite leg.

Chair Goddess Pose (Chair Utkata Konasana)

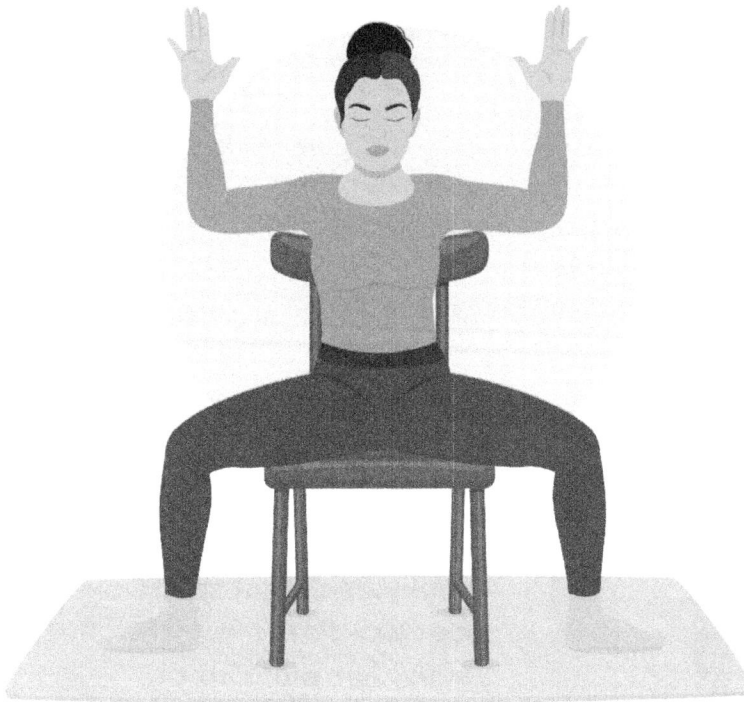

Chair Goddess pose works out your hips, arms, and inner thighs. It is helpful in gaining flexibility of the inner thigh muscles and strength in the arms.

Step-by-Step Instructions

- Sit up tall and comfortable towards the edge of the chair with your spine erect and relaxed, feet planted firmly on the floor at about hip-width apart.

- Rest your hands on your upper thighs just above your knees and take a deep breath in through your nose and slowly exhale.

- Widen your legs such that each leg gets to either side of the chair.

- Reach your arms out to the side, stretch them widely while keeping the fingertips engaged, and bend your elbows at about a 90-degree angle with palms facing forward.

- Hold this position for 5-10 deep breaths.

- Gently bring your legs back and arms down to release the pose.

- Repeat.

Cross-Legged Side Bend

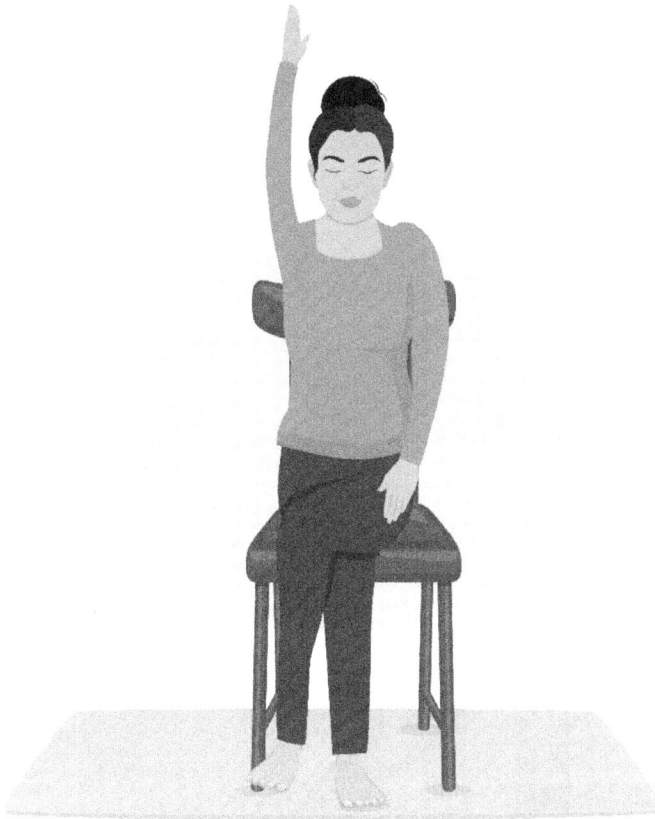

This pose utilizes your arms, thighs, and obliques. It is very helpful in stretching, strengthening, and lengthening your torso and thighs.

Step-by-Step Instructions

• Sit up tall and comfortable towards the edge of the chair with your spine erect and relaxed, feet planted firmly on the floor at about hip-width apart.

• Rest your hands on your upper thighs just above your knees and take a deep breath in through your nose and slowly exhale.

• Bring your right leg on top of your left leg and place your left hand on your right thigh.

• Lift your right arm up above your head and bend over to the left, stretching the right side of your upper half.

• Ensure that both of your sitz bones remain planted on the chair seat.

• Hold this position for 5-10 deep breaths.

• Slowly lower your hand and leg to return to starting position.

• Repeat on the opposite side.

Warrior II (Virabhadrasana II)

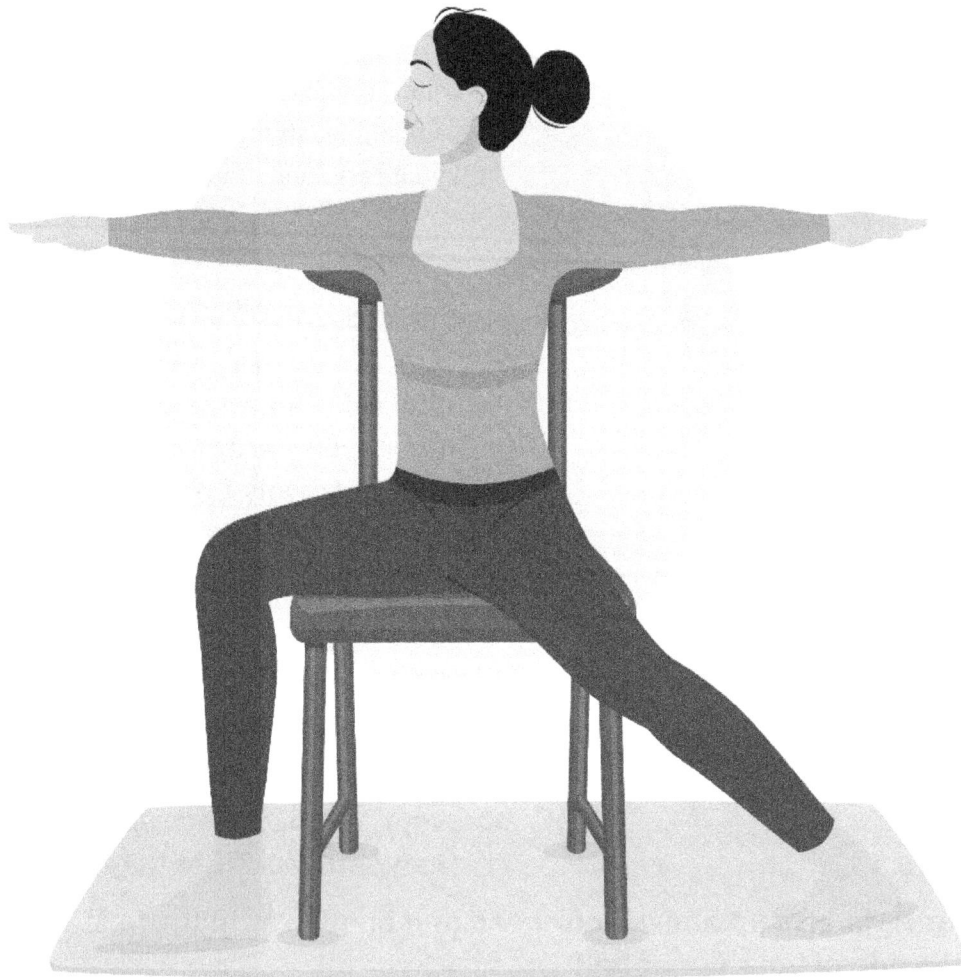

This pose helps work your legs, buttocks, hips, abs, thighs, and even arms. In this pose, your torso stays even so as to remind you that you shouldn't hang too far back. You may try Virabhadrasana II if you need some confidence, want to focus, or feel unstable and want to strengthen your lower half and become stable.

- Begin by sitting up tall towards the edge of the chair with your butt in the middle of the seat, so that you can easily pivot to the left and sit on your right side.

- Take a deep breath in through your nose and exhale slowly.

- Shift your body gently in a way that your right hamstring is flat on the seat of the chair with your right knee bent and straighten out your left leg and extend it back behind you.

- Keep your left foot angled out slightly more than in warrior I with the ankle farther back than the toes.

- Ensure that you can feel your feet planted on the ground firmly. Use your outer hips for control such that the bent knee is kept tracking forward and not rolling inward or off the chair.

- Use the back leg and outer foot to press firmly until you feel the weight in the inner left thigh.

- Ensure that your hips are kept even in the chair with your torso directly above them throughout the pose.

- Extend both of your hands straight out to the sides with palms facing down.

- Look over your right hand and keep your gaze above it.

- Hold there for 5-10 deep inhales and exhales.

- Bring your body back to the center of the chair slowly and in a gentle manner.

- Do the same for the opposite side.

- Repeat alternating the sides.

Quad Stretch

This pose stretches your quad muscles and hip flexors.

Step-by-Step Instructions

- Begin by standing behind a chair and holding its back with your right hand for support and balance.

- Grab the front of your left foot with your left hand and gently pull the heel towards your butt. Ensure to lift your chest up, push your hips forward to get a good hip flexor stretch, and engage your quadriceps.

- Hold the pose for about ten to twenty seconds then repeat switching the legs

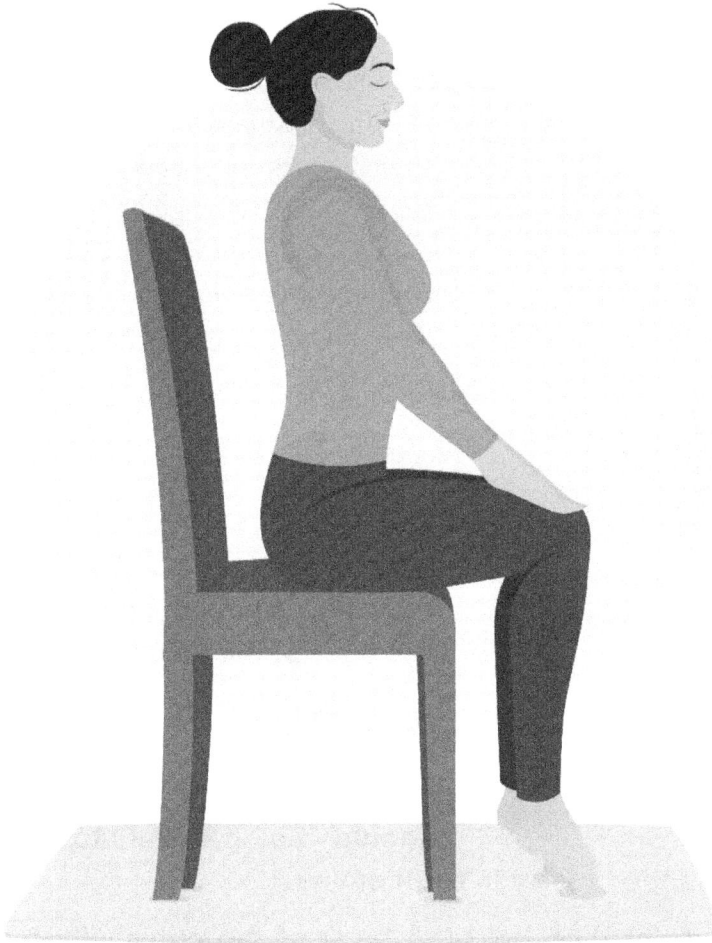

This pose engages your ankles, calves, toes, and shins. Pointing and flexing your feet helps stretch and strengthen your feet and ankles. It is also helpful if you want to work out any kinks from uncomfortable shoes.

Step-by-Step Instructions

- **Sit up tall and comfortable towards the edge of the chair with your spine erect and relaxed.**

- **Rest your hands on your upper thighs just above your knees and take a deep breath in through your nose and slowly exhale.**

- Lift your feet off the floor.

- Breathe in and point your toes forward, then breath out and flex your feet from the ankle pulling your toes back towards your chin.

- Repeat alternating between inhaling as you flex the feet and exhaling as you point the toes

Calf Stretch

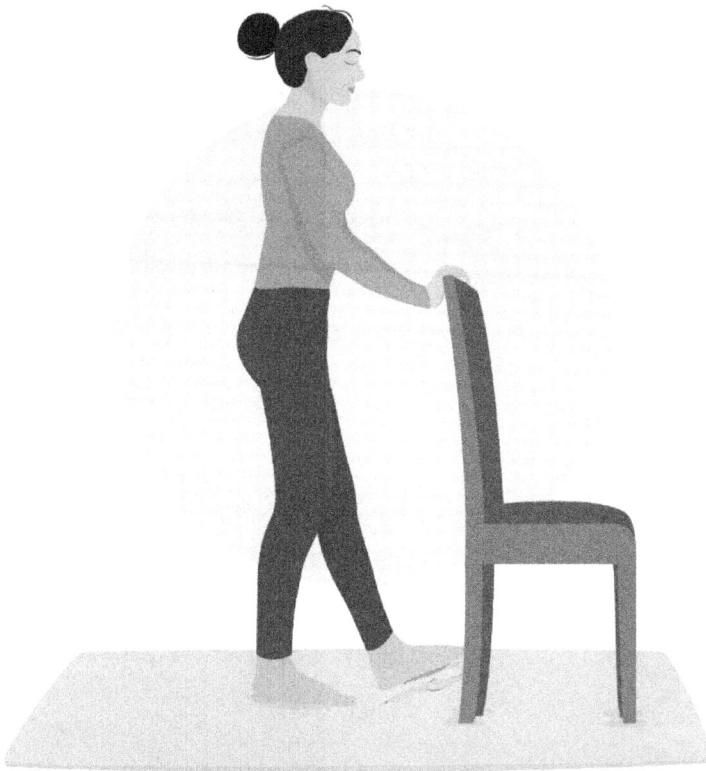

Just as the name suggests, calf stretch works out your calves. It helps stretch and strengthen the calf muscles and improves flexibility and mobility of your ankle joints which in turn improves your balance and stability.

Step-by-Step Instruction

- Place a bolster or a rolled-up blanket or towel on the floor behind a chair.

- Stand up tall behind the chair facing its back about a foot away from it. Your feet should be parallel to each other at hip-width apart and the bolster in front of you.

- Take a deep breath in and out then hold the back of the chair with both hands. Ensure that you feel stable and relaxed.

- Make a step forward with your right foot and place its ball on the bolster or folded blanket/towel. Ensure to keep the heel of the calf you are stretching on the floor and your hips back and over the heel. Hold this position for a few breaths.

- Release and do the same to your left leg.

- Repeat alternating the legs.

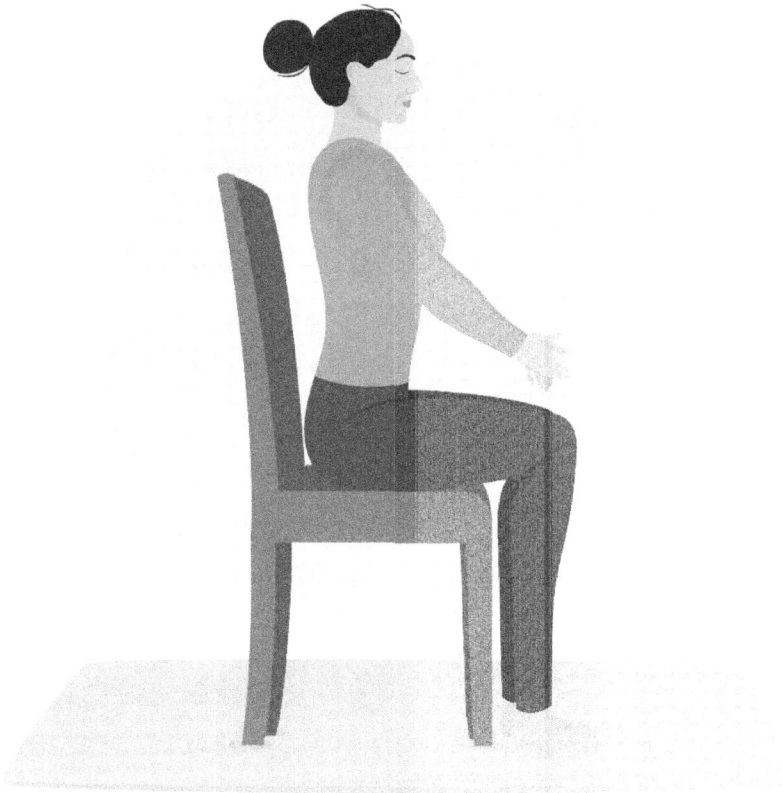

Palming

- Sit tall and comfortable in your chair

- Bring your palms together and rub them against each other until you feel warmth in them

- Cup them slightly and gently place them over your face covering your eyes. You may close your eyes or keep them open.

- Feel the warmth of the palms on your eyes. Ensure not to put pressure on your eyeballs.

- Hold the pose for about three to five minutes.

Cooling Breath (Sithali)

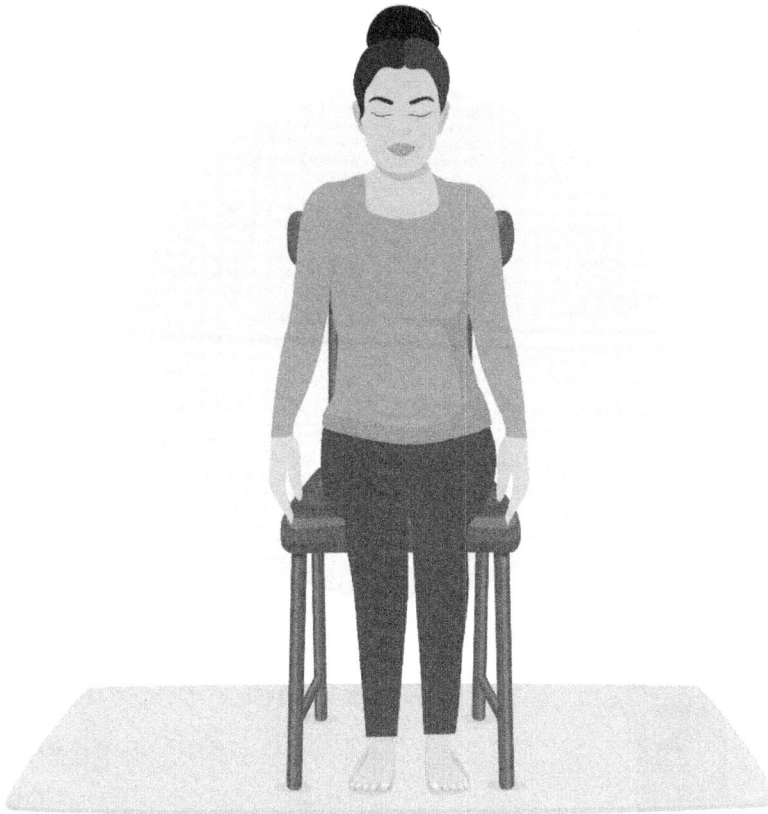

- Sit up tall in the chair with your hips towards the edge of the chair, back straight, your feet planted firmly on the floor at a hip-width apart.

- Place your palms face-down on your thighs.

- Take deep breaths in and out twice or thrice through your nose to prepare for this pranayama.

- Curl the sides of your tongue inwards towards the center to roll it into a tube-like shape. If you can't roll your tongue, purse your lips to make a small "o" shape with your mouth.

- Inhale slowly through the tube if you roll your tongue or channel the air through the "o" shaped opening if your lips are pursed.

- Close your mouth and breathe out slowly through your nose.

- Repeat until you feel the maximum cooling effect.

Final Relaxation and Meditation

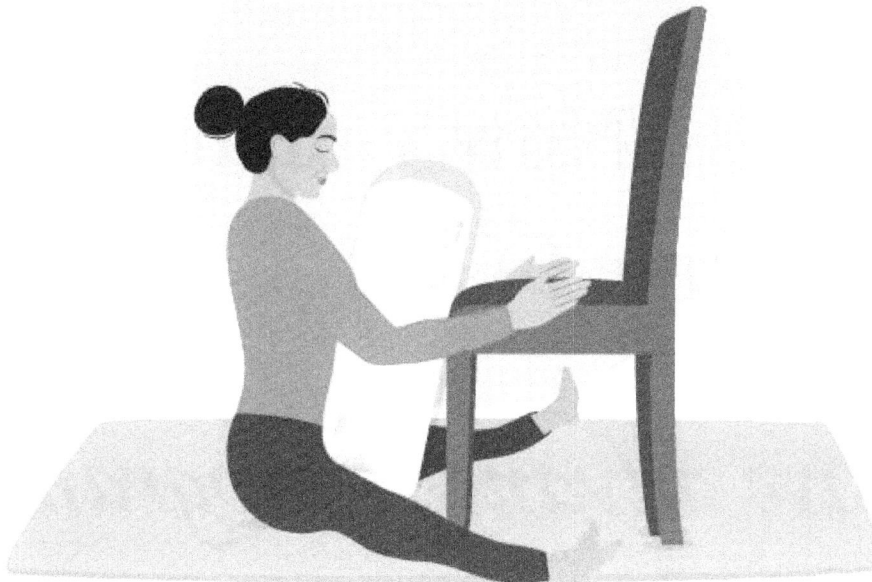

- Place a bolster on the chair seat
- Sit down on the ground facing the chair with your legs extended and straighten out under the chair.

- Ensure that you can easily reach the chair seat and rest your head on the bolster comfortably. If you can't, then sit on a block or something to raise you.

- Place your forehead on the bolster and hold the back of the chair by the sides with both hands and allow your entire body to relax.

- Close your eyes and become aware of your relaxed breathing. Pay attention to the relaxed inhales and exhales.

- After about three or five minutes, slowly open your eyes and gently lift your head.

Well done! Now you are ready to move to our

exclusive advanced program

Chapter Five:
Our Exclusive Advanced Program

Our exclusive advanced program consists of chair yoga workouts that are a bit advanced and more challenging than those in our intermediate program. However, they are still gentle for you so don't be scared of the word "advanced."

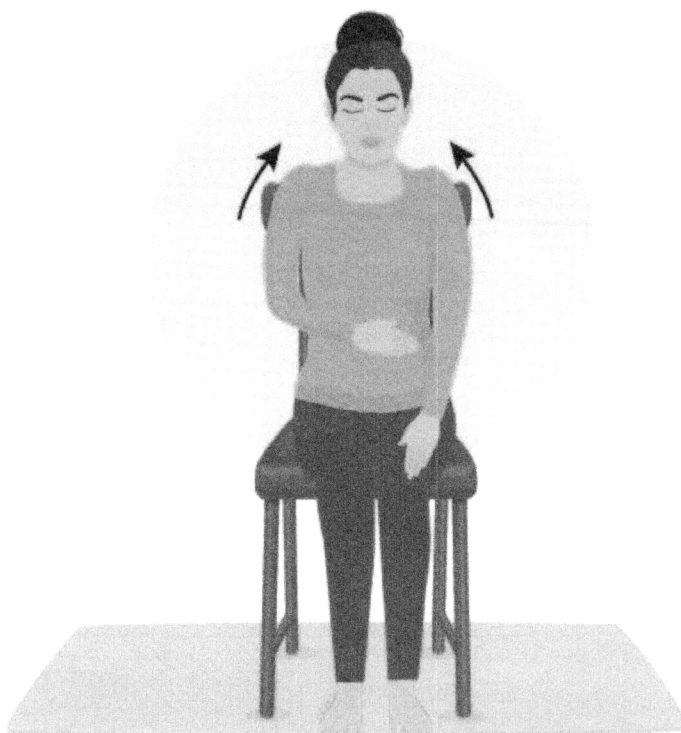

- Sit up tall in the chair with your hips towards the edge of the chair, back straight, your feet planted firmly on the floor at a hip-width apart.

- Place one hand on your belly and keep the other one resting on your thigh.

- Take a short forceful breath in followed by a short, sharp breath out.

- Do it over and over again for about one minute.

- On the last pump, take a break before you repeat the pumping.

Seated Head Circles

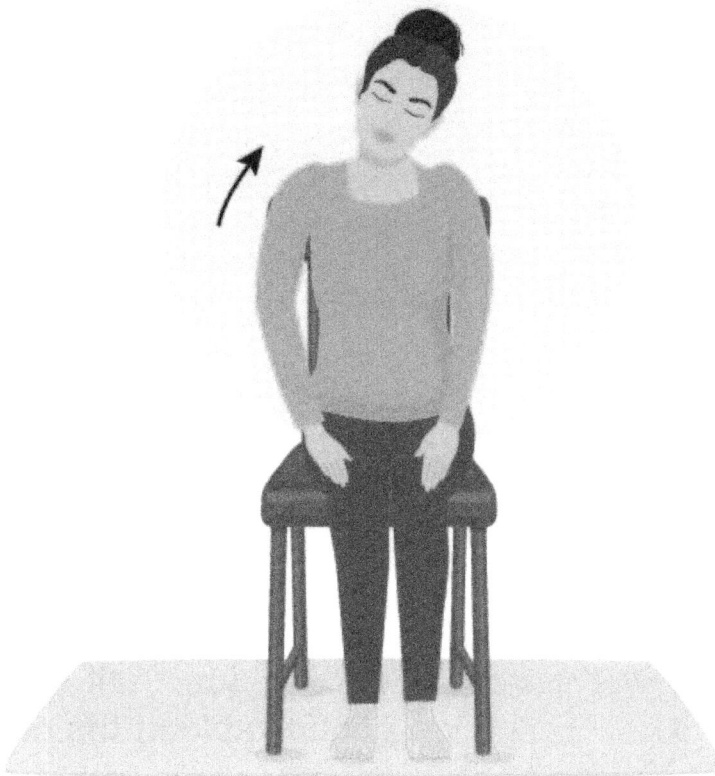

Being flexible in your upper neck and head opens you up for more creative thinking. Head circles help with this. Try them when you feel that you're not moving in your work and you need a little break or want to stimulate your thoughts.

Step-by-Step Instructions

- Sit up tall and comfortable at the edge of the chair with your spine erect and relaxed, feet flat on the floor at about hip-width apart.

- Rest your hands on your upper thighs just above your knees and take a deep breath in through your nose and slowly exhale.

- Try to imagine that you have an arrow on your nose and want to circle it clockwise.

- Begin making small circles and increase their size as your neck warms up.

- Move your head in a clockwise direction about 5-10 times.

- Circle it in an anticlockwise direction about 5-10 times.

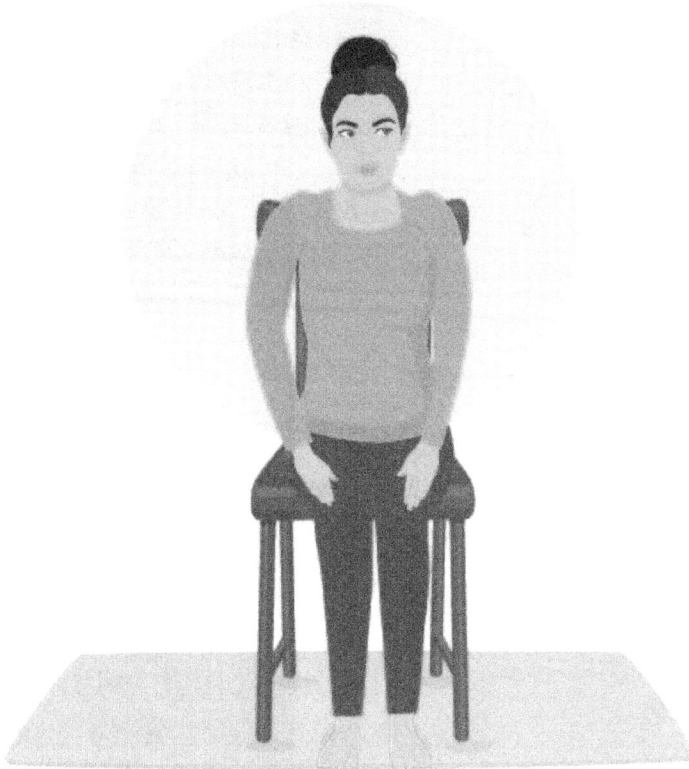

This movement is a great way to tease your mind. It might feel strange at first, but with time, it gets easier. Do this movement when you feel that your eyes are getting lazy, want to challenge them, or if you want to tease your mind and focus. Don't overdo the movement if you feel dizzy.

Step-by-Step Instructions

- Sit up tall and comfortable at the edge of the chair with your spine erect and relaxed, feet flat on the floor at about hip-width apart.

- Rest your hands on your upper thighs just above your knees and take a deep breath in through your nose and slowly exhale.

- Move your both eyes around 5 times in a clockwise direction, take a deep breath in and out then move them again 5 times in an anticlockwise direction.

- Repeat.

Sides-to-sides with Lower Jaw (Mouth Movement)

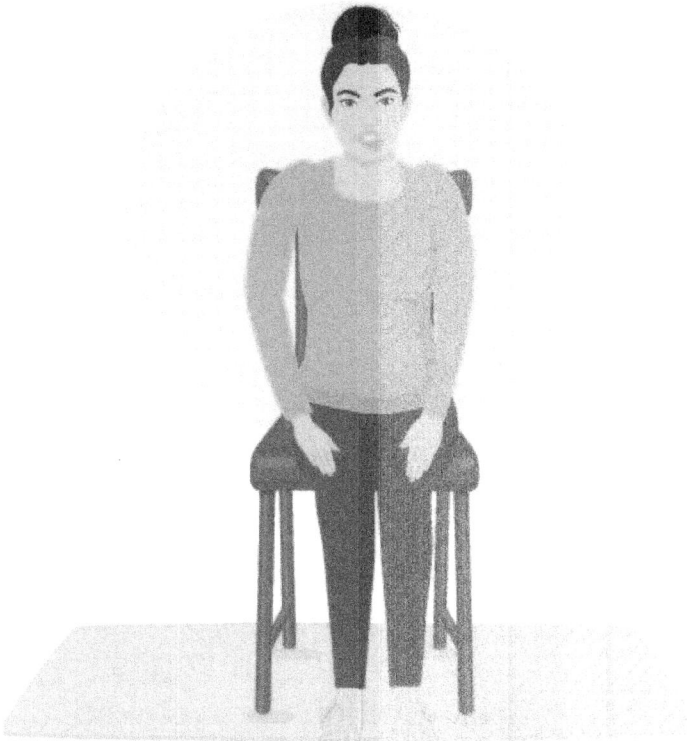

You can easily move your jaw around and find its mobility and range of motion. Most of us do not often stress our facial muscles. This movement helps release tension from the jaws and relieve anxiety.

Step-by-Step Instructions

- Sit up tall and comfortable at the edge of the chair with your spine erect and relaxed, feet flat on the floor at about hip-width apart.

- Rest your hands on your upper thighs just above your knees and take a deep breath in through your nose and slowly exhale.

- Relax your lower jaw and release it from your upper jaw, then move it from side to side.

- Repeat.

Shoulder Swings

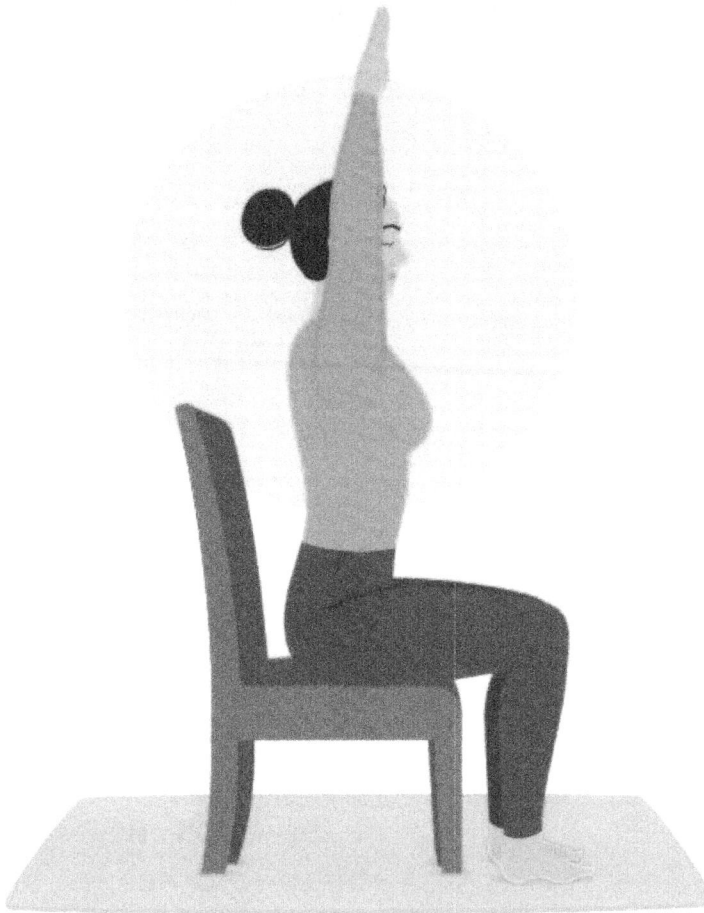

This move helps strengthen your shoulder muscles and improve the mobility of your shoulder joints.

Step-by-Step Instructions

- Sit upright in the chair so that your back isn't leaning on the chair
- Keep your feet flat and firmly planted on the floor at a hip distance apart with your palms on your thighs and shoulders relaxed.
- Drop your hands to the sides with your palms facing behind you
- Lift your arms up at shoulder height or higher
- Hold there for a few seconds then,
- Bring them back beside your hips
- Repeat.

High Altar Side Leans

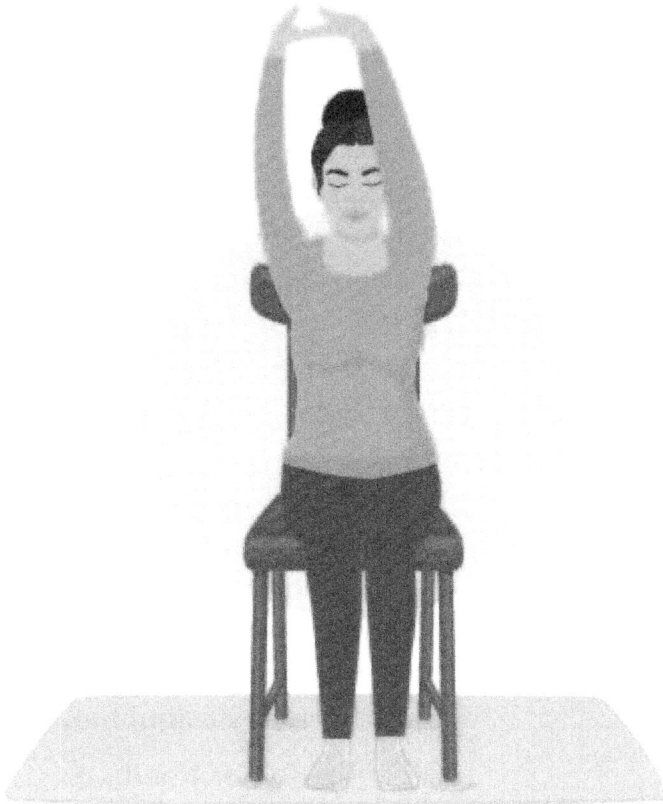

This exercise gives your arm and waist muscles a deeper stretch. It also helps open up your lungs and release tension in your shoulders and wrists.

Step-by-Step Instructions

- Sit up tall and comfortable towards the edge of the chair with your spine erect and relaxed, feet flat on the floor at about hip-width apart, and a straight back.

- Rest your hands on your upper thighs just above your knees and take a deep breath in through your nose and slowly exhale.

- Extend your arms straight out in front of you, interlace the fingers and keep the palms inverted such that they face away from your torso. Hold here for a few seconds and just feel the stretch.

- Keeping your ribs relaxed, raise your arms up above your head. Ensure that your shoulder tops remain down and stretch from elbow to wrist.

- Gently and slowly lean to the left as far as you can with your right hip still anchored to the chair seat. Hold here for 3-5 breaths and come back to the center.

- Then, lean over to the right and hold for 3-5 breaths.

- Repeat on each side.

Upside-Downside Finger Extensions

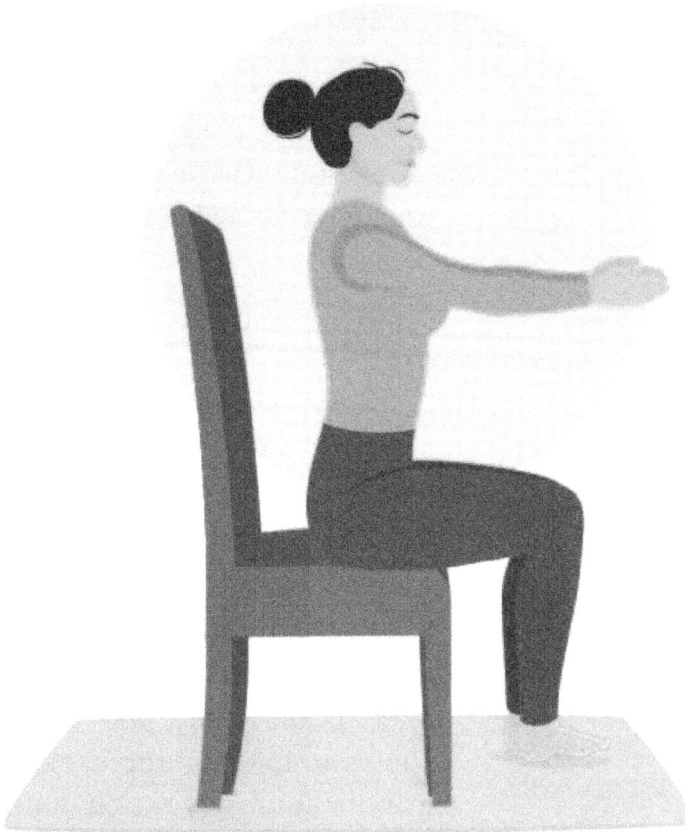

This finger movement works out your hands, shoulder, arms, and fingers. It strengthens the muscles in these areas. It also increases circulation in the hands and arms and helps improve flexibility and mobility of your shoulder and finger joints.

Step-by-Step Instructions

- Sit up tall and comfortable towards the edge of the chair with your spine erect and relaxed, feet flat on the floor at about hip-width apart, and a straight back.

- Rest your hands on your upper thighs just above your knees and take a deep breath in through your nose and slowly exhale.

- Extend both arms in front of you

- Turn your right palm up facing the ceiling and the left palm down facing the floor

- Spread your fingers wide, hold for a few seconds

- Then, close your fist into a ball and hold for a few seconds too

- Repeat alternating between spreading the fingers and closing them into a fistball.

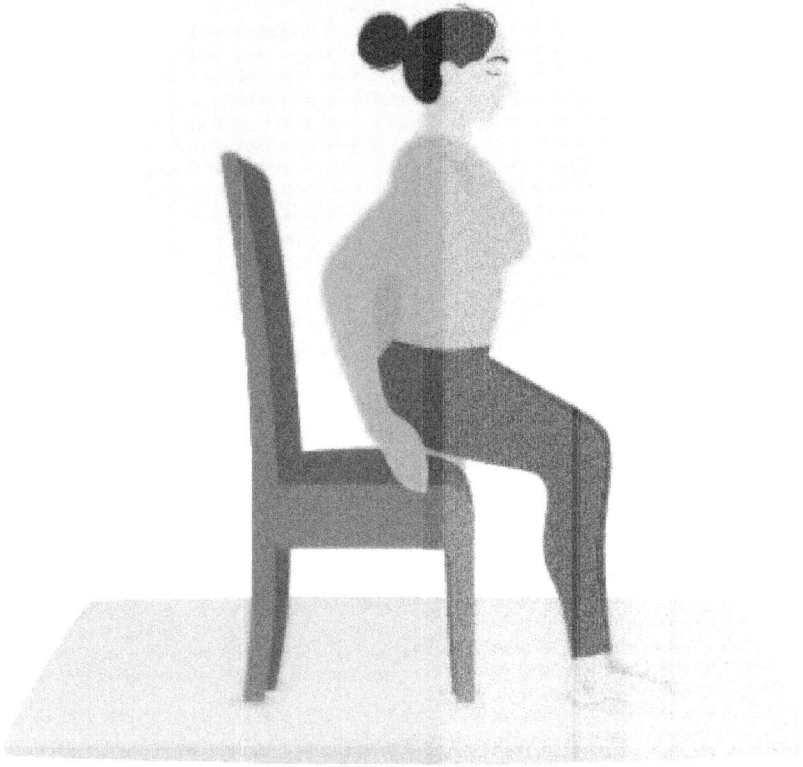

Seat Lifts

This exercise works out your transverse abdominals, pelvic floor muscles, and your core muscles. It helps stretch and strengthen these muscles. Try this out if you need to access your innermost abdominals and work them out.

Step-by-Step Instructions

- Sit up tall and comfortable towards the edge of the chair with your spine erect and relaxed, feet flat on the floor at about hip-width apart, and a straight back.

- Rest your hands on your upper thighs just above your knees and take a deep breath in through your nose and slowly exhale.

- Bring your hands and hold the edges of your chair seat.

- Relax for a second then slowly lift your butt up off the chair. Try as much as possible not to engage or use your legs.

- Imagine lifting yourself up using your arms and abdominals, and pressing your shoulders down. Hold there for a few breaths then slowly release the pose.

- Repeat.

Intense Side Stretch (Parsvottanasana)

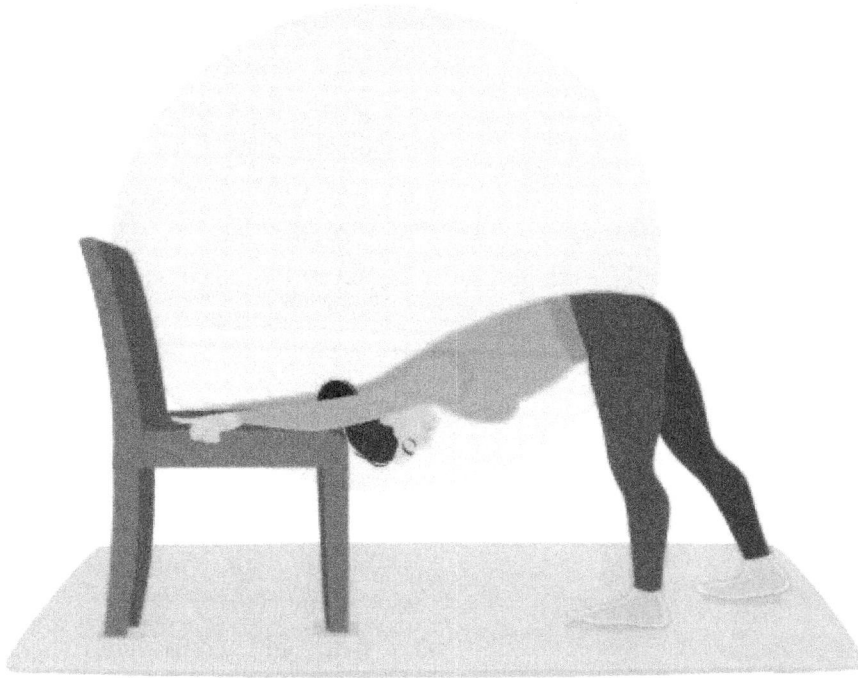

This pose engages the muscles of your shoulders, back, arms, hips, and legs. It is helpful in stretching and strengthening your legs and gaining flexibility in the hip muscles and mobility of your hip joint. Although this stretch may be intense at the beginning, it is very functional and can help you move more freely in daily life.

Step-by-Step Instructions

- Stand up tall in front of the chair facing it. Your feet should be parallel to each other at hip-width apart.

- Take a deep breath in and out then hold the chair seat with both hands. Ensure that you feel stable and relaxed.

- Make one step backward with your right foot and place it down at about a leg's length behind you or away from your left foot.

- Keep your back nice, relaxed, and lengthened, and both legs straight engaging the quadriceps and the area above the kneecaps.

- Keeping your back straight, slowly tilt your torso forward as if you are laying your chest over your front thigh until it is parallel to the ground.

- Hold this position for about 5-10 deep inhales and exhales

- Repeat for the opposite leg.

Chair Boat Pose (Chair Navasana)

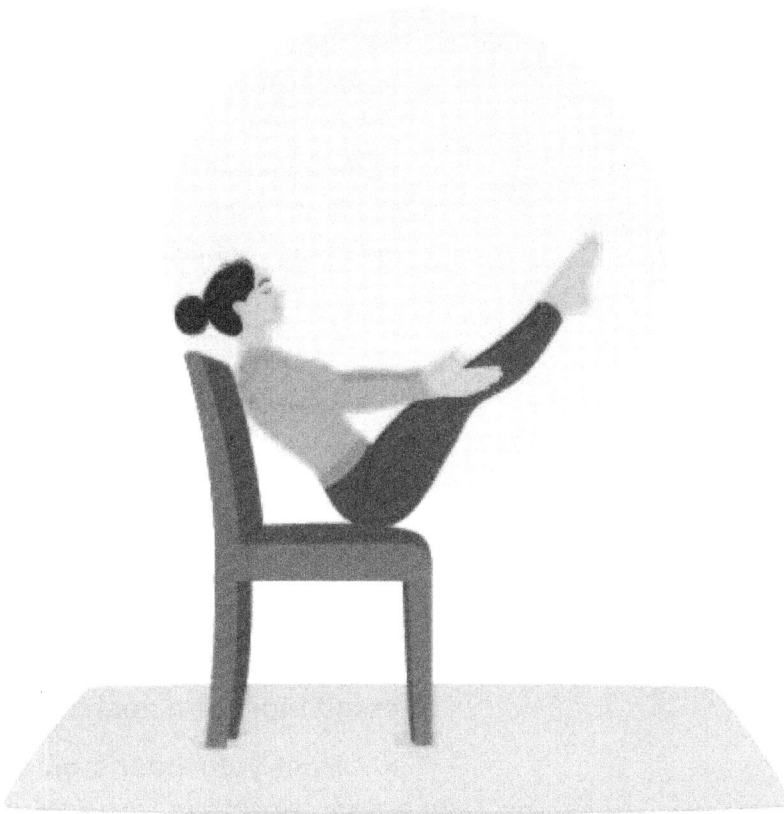

Chair Navasana works out the abdominals, hamstrings, hips, and quadriceps. Try it out if you want to strengthen these muscles.

Step-by-Step Instructions

- Sit up tall and comfortable towards the edge of the chair with your spine erect and relaxed, feet flat on the floor at about hip-width apart.

- Rest your hands on your upper thighs just above your knees and take a deep breath in through your nose and slowly exhale.

- Lean back engaging your abdominals and lift your legs off the ground with your feet flexed.

- Hold this position for about 3-5 deep breaths

- Gently release the legs back to the ground one at a time.

- Repeat.

Chair Goddess Twist (Chair Parivrtta Utkata Konasana)

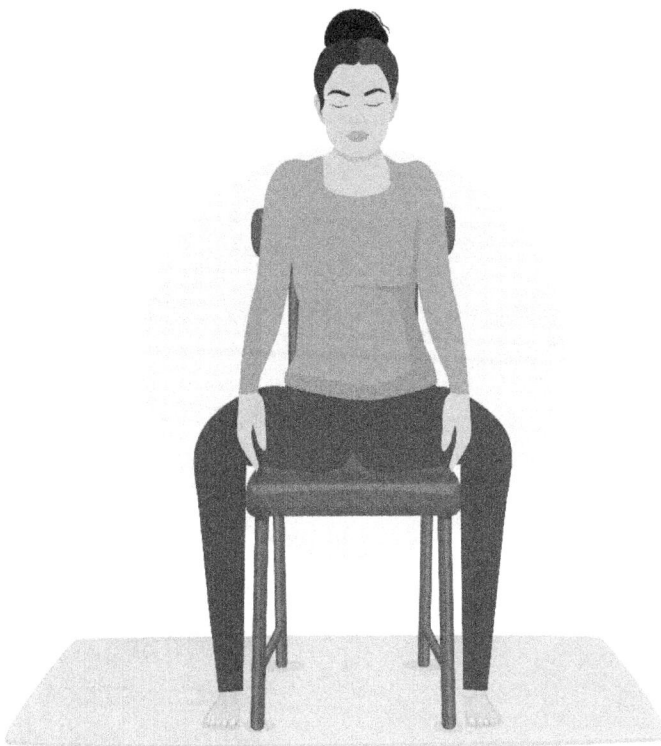

This pose engages and works out the sides of your torso, your inner thighs, arms, and hips. It is good for stretching and strengthening the oblique muscles and arms. It also helps boost your mood and confidence.

Step-by-Step Instructions

- Sit up tall and comfortable towards the edge of the chair with your spine erect and relaxed, feet planted firmly on the floor at about hip-width apart.

- Rest your hands on your upper thighs just above your knees and take a deep breath in through your nose and slowly exhale.

- Widen your legs such that each leg gets to either side of the chair.

- Slowly and gently twist your upper body towards the left, lifting your right arm up above your head and lowering your left arm down towards your left ankle with your palms facing forward.

- Look up towards your right hand and gaze at the palm

- Hold there for 5-10 deep breaths

- Gently bring your legs back and your right arms down to release the pose

- Repeat.

Warrior III (Virabhadrasana III)

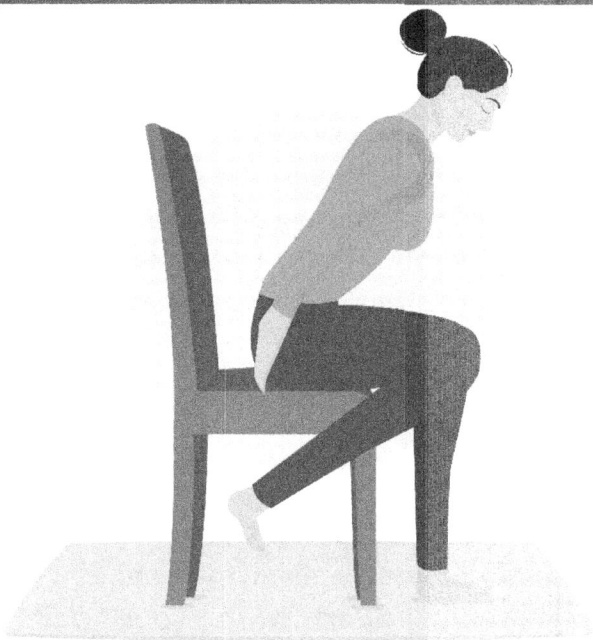

Chair warrior III is more challenging but super fun to perform. It requires you to have a lot of abdominal control and strength in the buttocks. You can perform this exercise when you are in need of some focus and energy or want to challenge your balance and improve it. This pose helps work out your buttocks, core, and back.

Step-by-Step Instructions

• Begin by sitting up tall towards the edge of the chair with your butt in the middle of the seat, so that you can easily pivot to the left and sit on your right side.

• Take a deep breath in through your nose and exhale slowly.

• Gently inch over towards the left side of the chair with your right hamstring flat on the seat of the chair, right knee bent and straighten out your left leg and extend it back behind you and ensure that your toes are pressed firmly on the floor.

• Bent forward until you can raise your back leg off the floor.

• Stretch your arms straight out to the sides with palms facing down. You can stretch your arms straight back too.

• Hold there for about 5-10 deep inhales and exhales.

• Repeat on the opposite side.

Cross-legged Twist

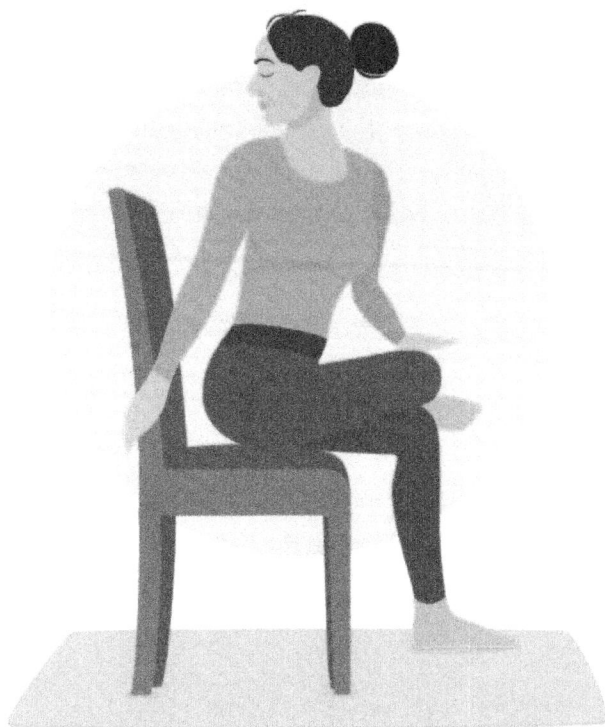

This pose engages the back, legs, and hips. It is helpful in gaining muscle flexibility and joint mobility in the spine and hips. It also helps relieve tension and stiffness. Thanks to its twisting motion.

Step-by-Step Instructions

- Sit up tall in the chair leaving some space behind you. Plant your feet flat and firmly on the floor at a hip distance apart with your palms facing down on the upper side of your thighs.

- Take a deep breath in and out then bring your entire right leg and cross it on top of your left thigh.

- Let your left hand rest on your right thigh as the right hand rest on the chair seat behind you

- Breathe in as you lengthen your spine, then breathe out and twist your upper body towards the right. Look behind and go as far as you can.

- Hold there for 3-5 deep breaths.

- Unwind from the twist slowly and gently, returning to the center and uncrossing your leg, putting it back on the floor.

- Repeat for the opposite side.

Advanced Hamstring Stretch

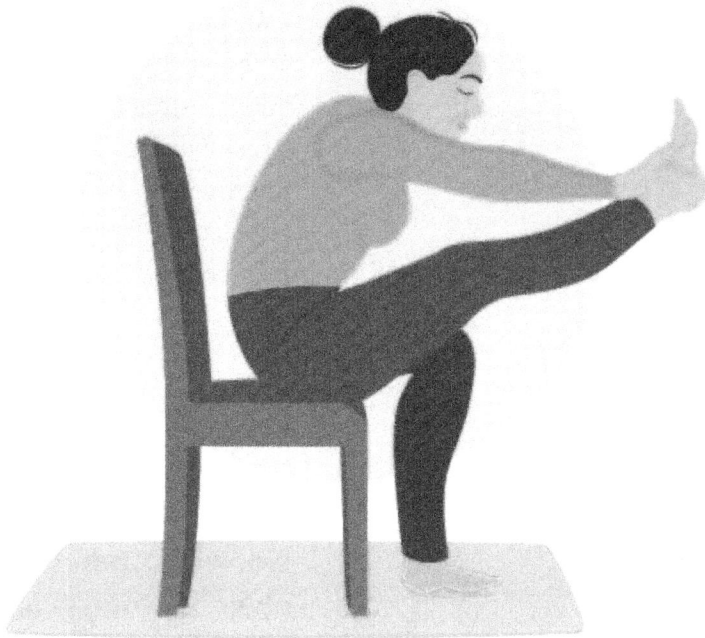

This stretch is quite intense but good for you. Not only does it open up your entire back but it also engages your core and lower back. Advanced hamstring stretch works out your hamstrings, abs, arms, and legs. It is the best exercise for stretching your hamstrings, inner thighs, and legs.

Step-by-Step Instructions

- Sit up tall and comfortable towards the edge of the chair with your spine erect and relaxed, feet flat on the floor at about hip-width apart.

- Rest your hands on your upper thighs just above your knees and take a deep breath in through your nose and slowly exhale.

- Hold your right ankle and straighten your leg out in front of you. Hold the pose for about 3-5 deep breaths.

- Now, try lifting the leg up towards your face, while maintaining a straight back. Hold for another 3-5 deep breaths.

- Sit upright again and try to open the leg to the right side for another 3-5 deep breaths

- For a hamstring and IT band stretch, bring the leg across the midsection and then to the left. Hold this position for another 3-5 deep breaths then release the leg.

- Repeat for the opposite leg.

High Lunge

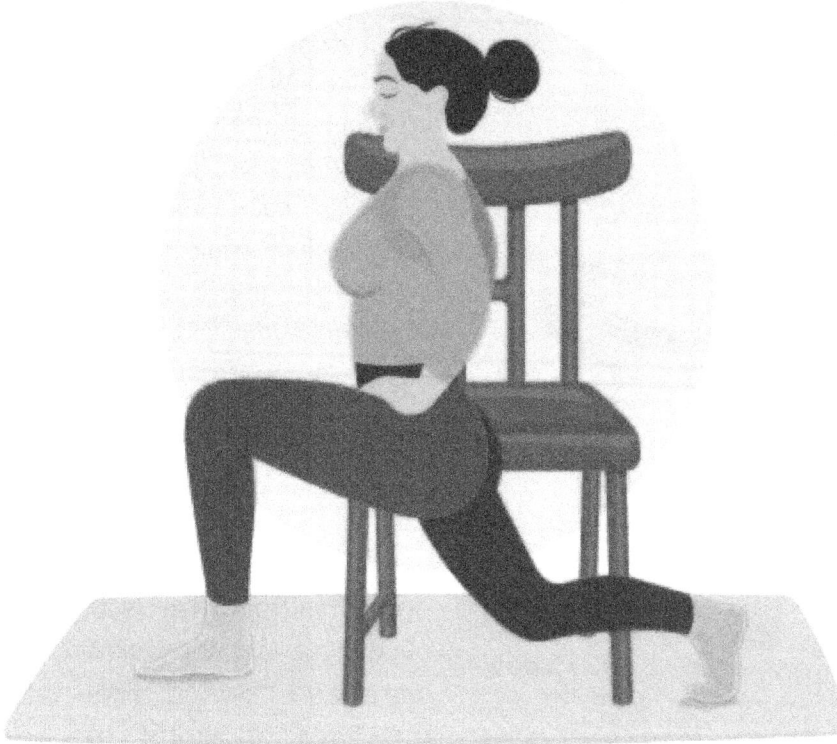

This pose works out your quads, hips, hamstrings, and glutes. It is good for deep full-body stretching and strengthening. It improves blood circulation and boosts metabolism.

Step-by-Step Instructions

- Stand up tall sideways behind a chair. Your feet should be parallel to each other at hip-width apart.

- Take a deep breath in and out then hold on to the chair back with your right hand and make a leg's length step backward with your left leg.

- Lunge the right knee deeply until the thigh becomes almost parallel to the chair seat.

- Ensure to keep the knee above the ankle to protect it.

- Press through your left knee firmly and extend your left knee behind. Keep your right glute muscles and abdominals deeply engaged and anchor the whole right foot to the ground. Lift your left hand up towards the ceiling.

- Hold there for about 5-10 deep breaths

- Return to an upright standing position and repeat for the opposite leg.

Tree

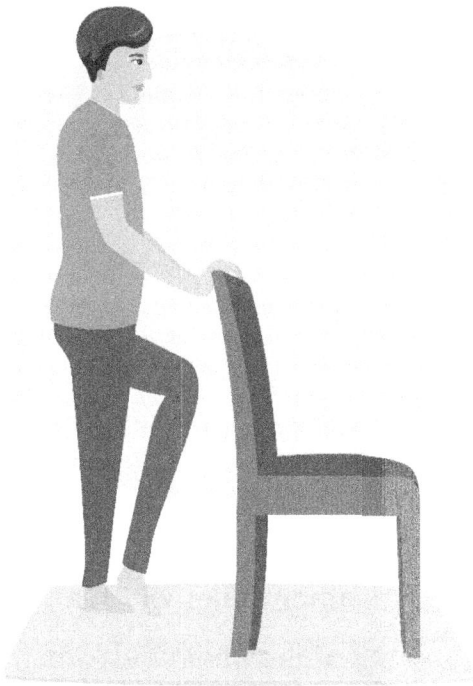

Tree pose works your hips and legs. It helps stretch and strengthen the muscles of the standing leg and improve mobility and flexibility of the hip joint. This exercise also helps improve body awareness and balance.

Step-by-Step Instructions

- Stand up tall sideways behind a chair. Your feet should be parallel to each other at hip-width apart.

- Take a deep breath in and out then hold on to the chair back with your left hand.

- Place your right hand on your hip and bend your right knee.

- Let your right heel rest on your left leg while the toes of your right foot touch the floor.

- Try to move your right foot up such that its sole rests on your left leg just below the knee

- Once you feel stable, put your hands together in front of your chest. You can also try to lift them up or put them together above your head.

- Hold here for a few relaxed breaths

- Repeat with your opposite leg.

Raised Knee Balance

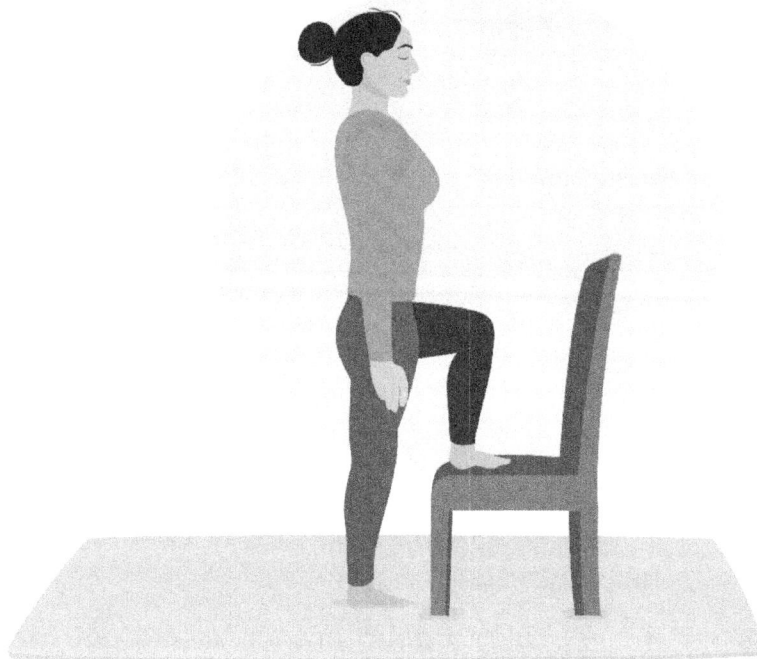

This posture works your hips, knee joints, and legs. It helps improve flexibility and mobility of the hip and knee joints. It also strengthens your leg muscles thus improving your stability and balance.

Step-by-Step Instruction

- Stand up tall in front of the chair with its side facing you. Your feet should be parallel to each other at hip-width apart.

- Take a deep breath in and out then hold the back of the chair with one hand for support. Ensure that you feel stable and relaxed.

- Slowly and mindfully lift the leg that is closest to the chair and put its foot on top of the chair seat. Ensure that your whole foot is on the seat.

- Hold here for a few relaxed breaths. You may try lifting your hand an inch off the chair if you feel your balance is good.

- You may also use a block for placing the foot if the chair is too high and just use the chair for support to hold onto.

- Slowly and gently return the leg to the floor and do the same with the other leg.

- Repeat, alternating the legs.

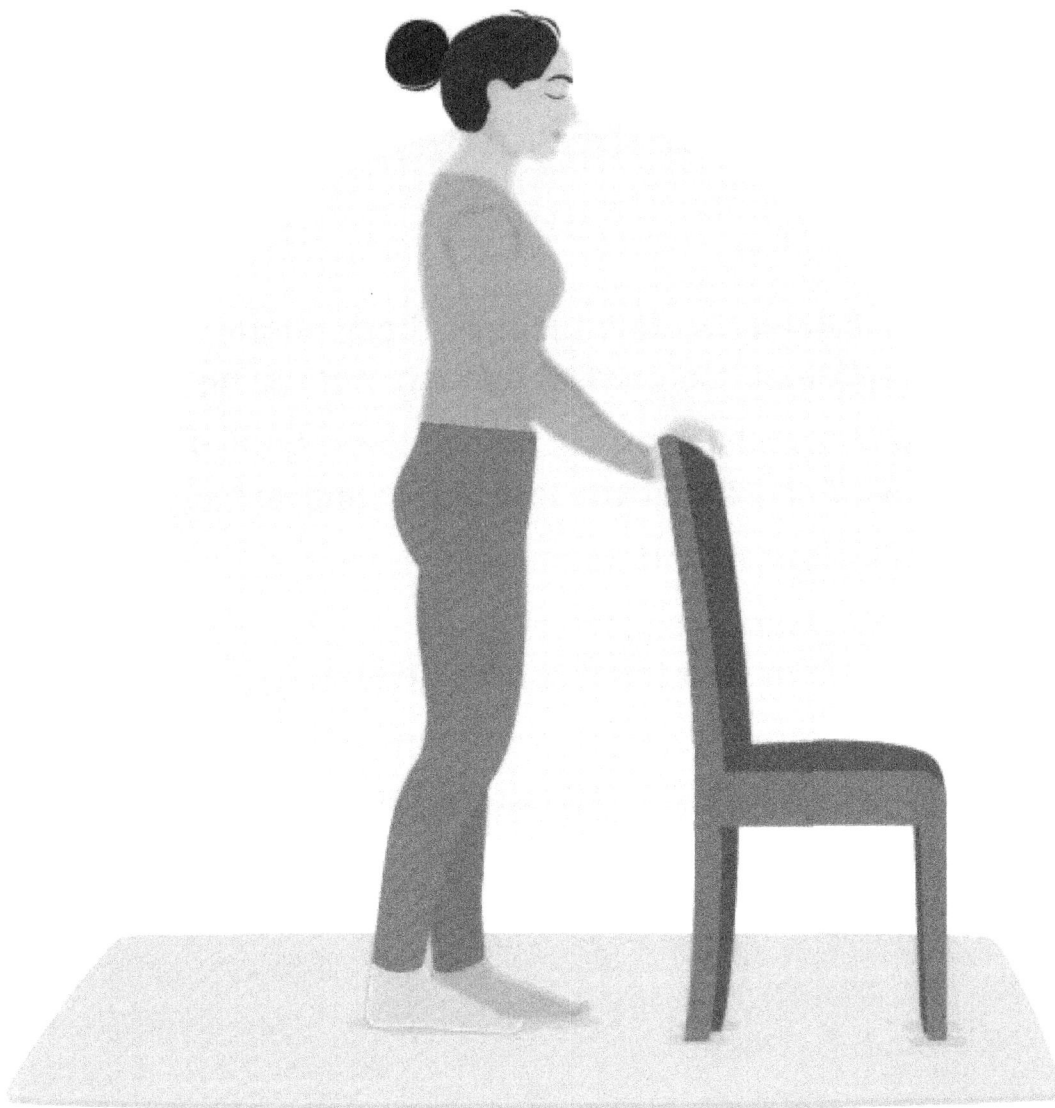

This pose will work out your feet, ankle, and calves. It helps strengthen your calf muscles, improve ankle joints and feet flexibility and mobility and improve balance and stability.

Step-by-Step Instruction

- Stand up tall behind a chair facing its back about a foot away from it. Your feet should be parallel to each other at hip-width apart.

- Take a deep breath in and out then hold the back of the chair with both hands. Ensure that you feel stable and relaxed.

- Rise onto the tips of your toes.

- Slowly lower your heels to the ground. Ensure that you don't feel any impact when your heels touch the floor.

- Raise your heels again and lower them in the same way.

- Repeat raising and lowering your heels as slowly and as quietly as possible

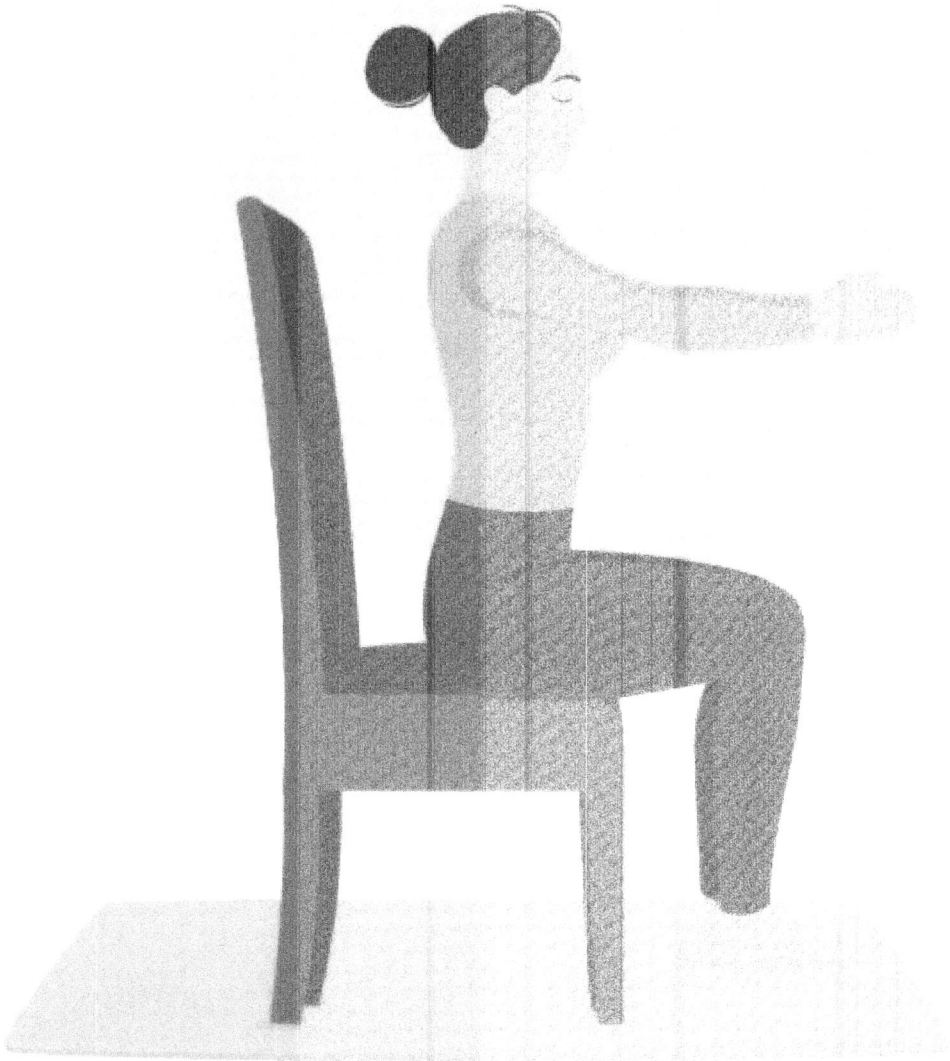

- Sit tall and comfortable in your chair

- Bring your palms together and rub them against each other until you feel warmth in them

- Cup them slightly and gently place them over your face covering your eyes. You may close your eyes or keep them open.

- Feel the warmth of the palms on your eyes. Ensure not to put pressure on your eyeballs.

- Hold the pose for about three to five minutes.

Cooling Breath (Sitkari)

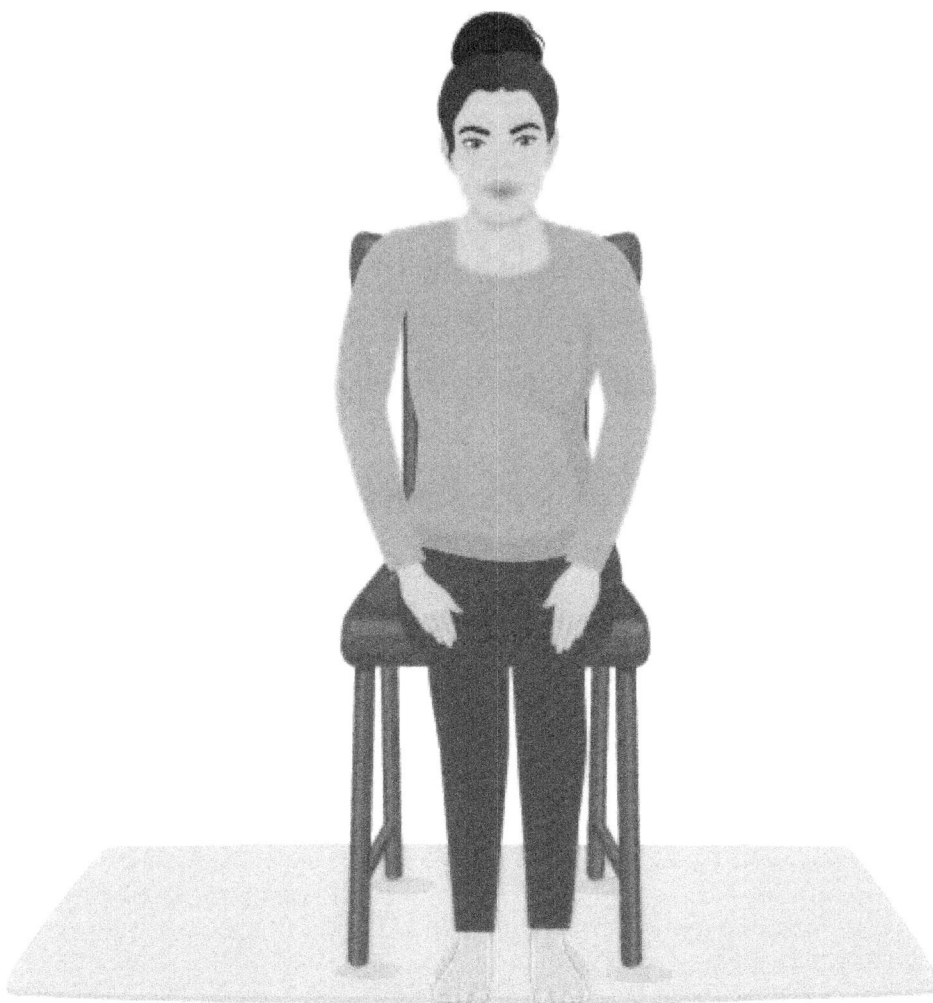

Sit up tall in the chair with your hips towards the edge of the chair, back straight, your feet planted firmly on the floor at a hip-width apart.

- **Take a few natural breaths in and out to center yourself.**

- **With your lips open, close your teeth by bringing your lower and upper teeth together and inhale through them producing a soft hissing sound.**

- **Release the teeth and close your mouth as you breathe out through the nose**

- **Repeat until you feel a nice cooling effect that eases your body and mind.**

Sit up tall and comfortable at the edge of the chair with your spine erect and relaxed, feet flat on the floor at about hip-width apart. Raise your feet using a bolster or a folded blanket if they can't

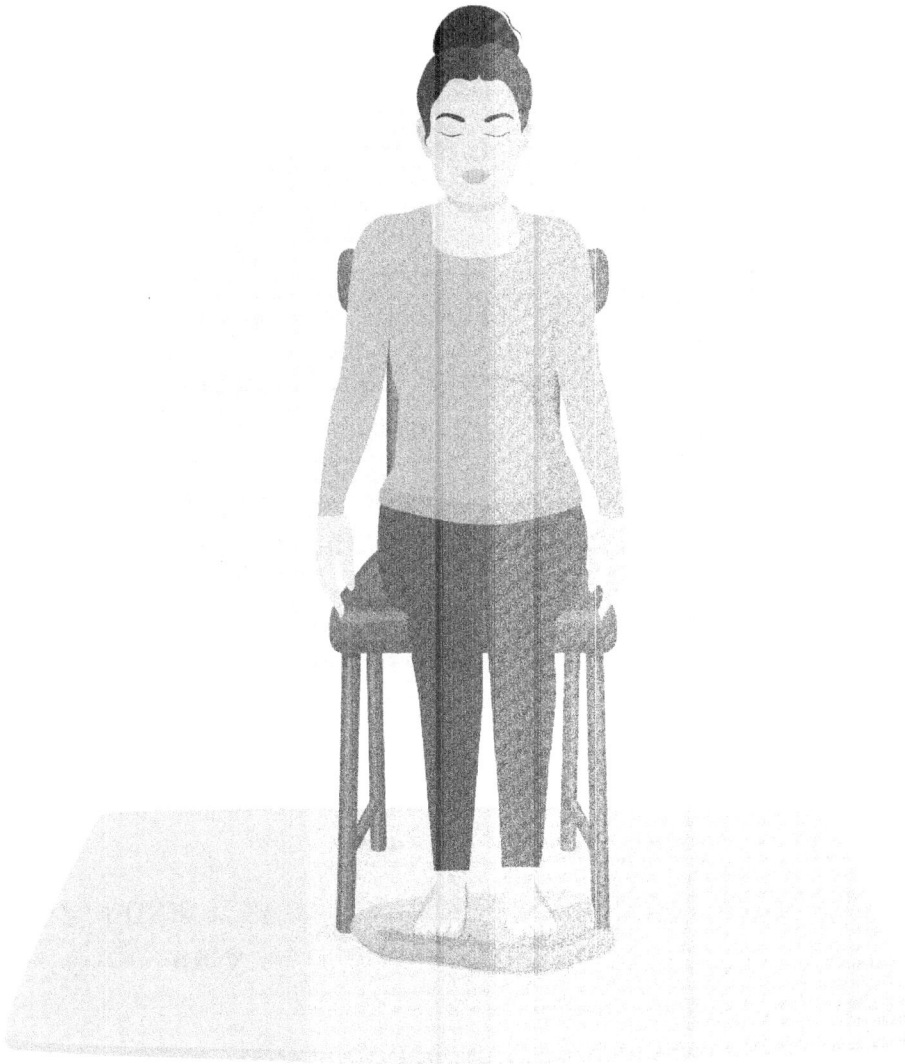

touch the ground when seated.

- Rest your hands on your upper thighs just above your knees and relax your entire body.

- Close your eyes and imagine a vibrant beautiful rainbow in the sky. It is so close that you can see all of its colors perfectly.

- Take a deep breath and as you inhale, visualize the color red. Keep your body relaxed and let go of any tension as you exhale.

- Take a deep breath and as you inhale, visualize the color orange. Breathe out and let go of any negative emotions.

- Take a deep breath and as you inhale, visualize the color yellow. Breathe out and relax your mind.

- Take a deep breath and as you inhale, visualize the color green. Breathe out and find a state of tranquility within yourself.

- Take a deep breath and as you inhale, visualize the color blue. Breathe out and fill yourself with love.

- Take a deep breath and as you inhale, visualize the color Indigo. Breathe out and locate your most hidden inner self.

- Take a deep breath and as you inhale, visualize the color violet. Breathe out and stay with your most intimate self.

- You are now on your deepest mental level.

- Now focus on any goal that you want to achieve in your workout or life. Be inspired by yourself.

- Prepare to come out from meditation. As you come out, you will feel a sense of peace and cleansing and your body will be in perfect harmony and ready to act.

Chapter Six:
Beginner Program for Osteoarthritis of the Hands, Knees, and Hips

Osteoarthritis is a common illness among senior adults. At least one out of three adults aged sixty and above are affected. Osteoarthritis is characterized by pain, stiffness, and swelling in the joints. The most frequently affected parts are the hips, hands, and knees.

When you keep aching joints active, they become less painful. And chair yoga is one of the best ways for affected seniors who are afraid of other strenuous and challenging exercises. Yoga moves help lubricate your joints, strengthen the muscles that support the joints, and prevent tendons and muscles from stiffening.

Exercises that involve a range of motion or rather flexibility exercises and strengthening exercises are the most important for people with ostcoarthritis. In this chapter, you will find gentle chair yoga poses that help with improving flexibility in your joints as well as strengthen your muscles. As usual, you need to prepare your mind and the breathing system since you will be breathing throughout the exercises. Let's get started.

Breathing Exercise

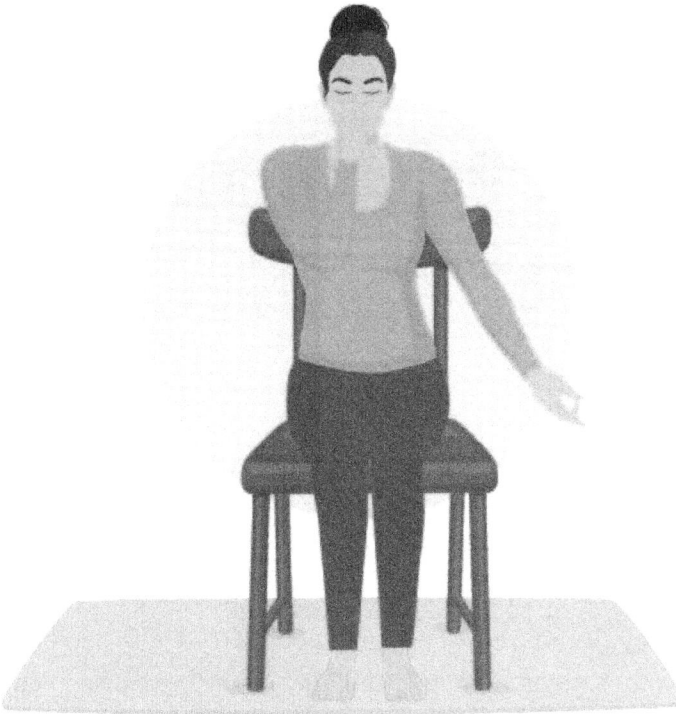

- Sit up tall and comfortable at the edge of the chair with your spine erect and relaxed, feet flat on the floor at about hip-width apart. Raise your feet using a bolster or a folded blanket if they can't touch the ground when seated. Rest your hands on your upper thighs just above your knees

- Place your right thumb on your right nostril and your ring finger or right forefinger on the left nostril. Maintain light contact with them throughout the breathing exercise.

- Close your right nostril by pressing it gently with the thumb and inhale through the left nostril.

- Release your thumb and close your left nostril by gently pressing it with your right forefinger or ring finger and breathe out through your right nostril.

- Keep your left nostril closed and breathe in through your right nostril

- Release your forefinger or ring finger on your left nose and close your right nose by gently pressing your right thumb and breathe out through your left nostril.

- This makes up one round. Perform another two rounds.

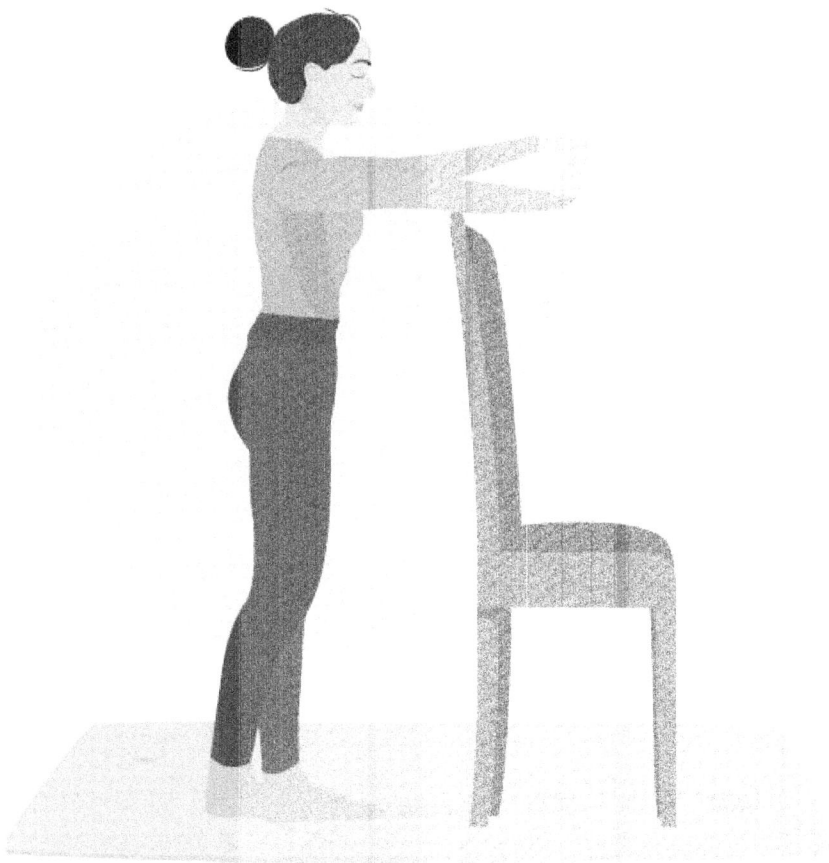

This exercise helps relieve cramping and achiness in your fingers, forearms, and wrists. It also helps relieve anxiety and keeps your mind focused.

Step-by-Step Instructions

- Sit up tall and comfortable towards the edge of the chair with your spine erect and relaxed, feet flat on the floor at about hip-width apart, and a straight back.

- Rest your hands on your upper thighs just above your knees and take a deep breath in through your nose and slowly exhale.

- Extend your right arm straight out in front of you with palms facing down.

- Bring your left arm and pull the right hand fingers back towards the torso. Hold there for a few breaths as you pull the fingers.

- Now, turn your right arm such that the palms face down, bring your left hand over it and press its back down. Hold for a few breaths.

- Lastly, turn the right palm up to face the ceiling and use your left hand to pull its fingers down holding for a few breaths.

- Repeat alternating the hands.

Finger Extensions

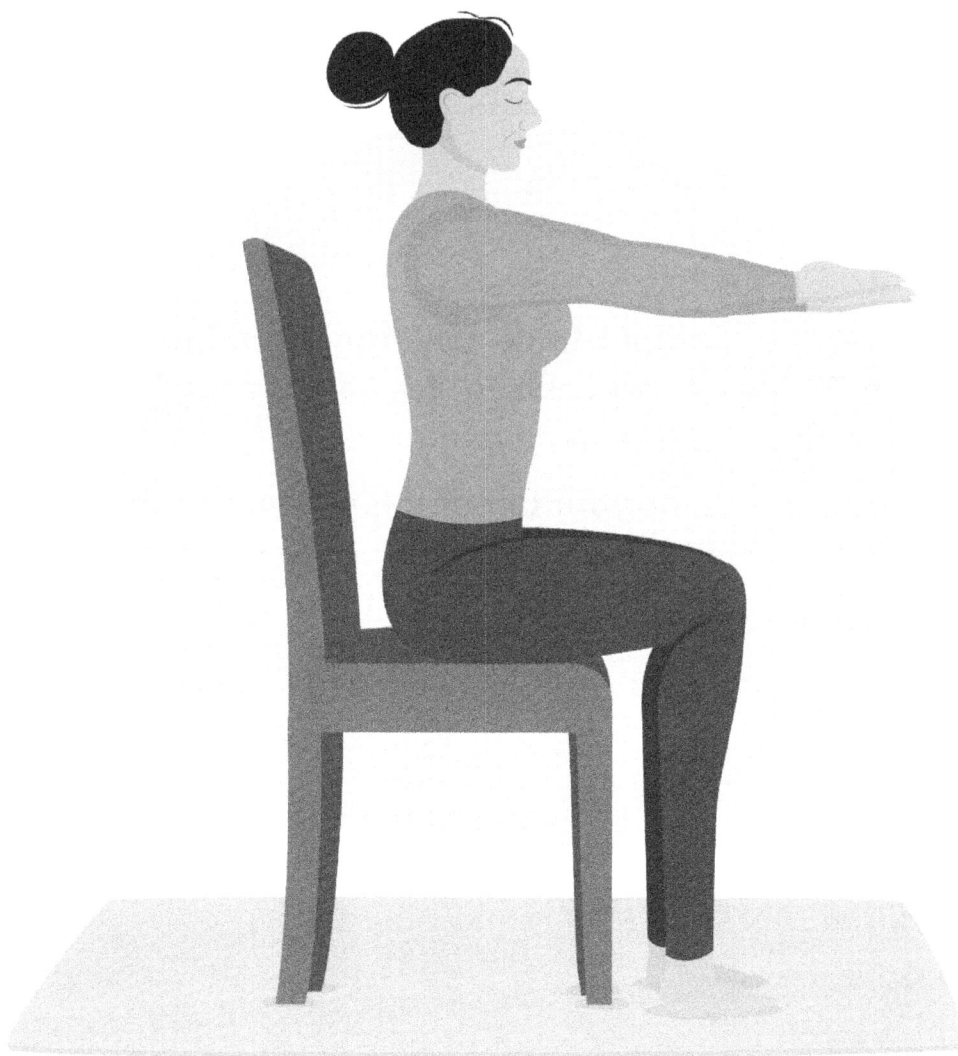

This exercise helps stretch your fingers and helps strengthen your hand, arms, and shoulder muscles. It also increases circulation in the hands and arms and helps improve flexibility and mobility of your finger joints.

Step-by-Step Instructions

- Sit up tall and comfortable towards the edge of the chair with your spine erect and relaxed, feet flat on the floor at about hip-width apart, and a straight back.

- Rest your hands on your upper thighs just above your knees and take a deep breath in through your nose and slowly exhale.

- Extend both arms in front of you

- Spread your fingers wide, hold for a few seconds

- Then, close your fist into a ball and hold for a few seconds too

- Repeat alternating between spreading the fingers and closing them into a fistball.

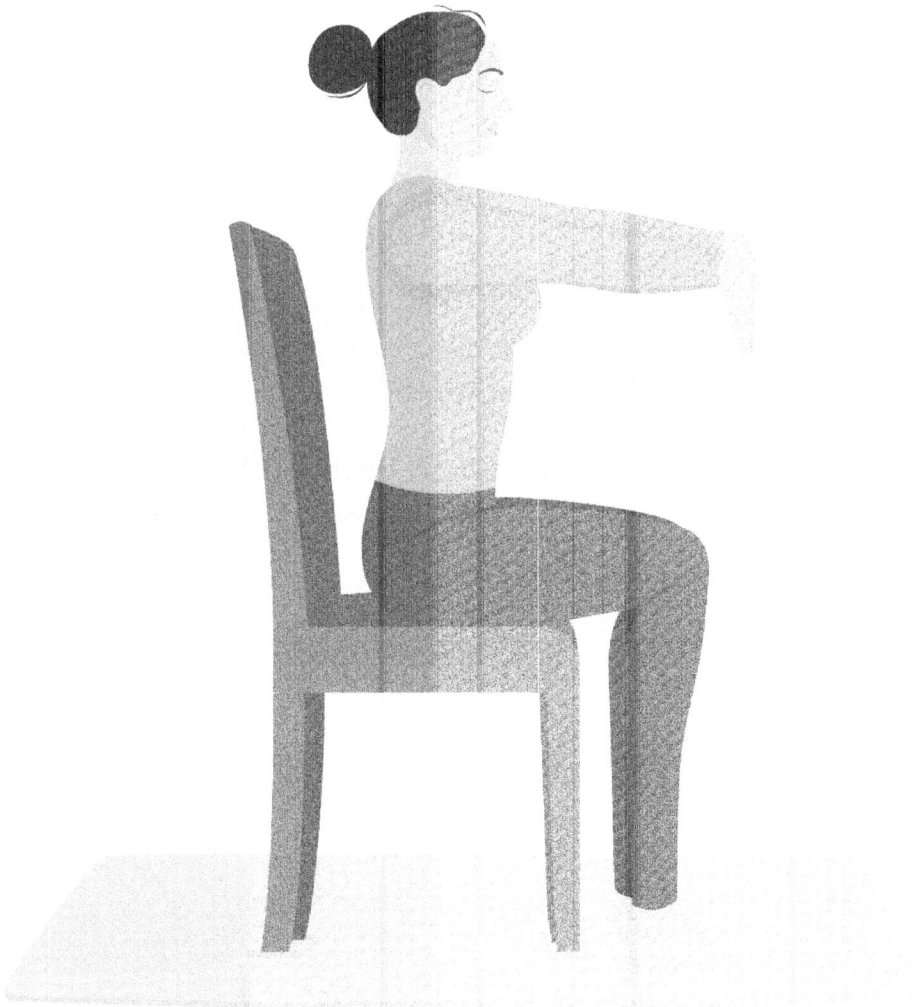

Wrist extensions work out your wrists, hands, and shoulders. They help strengthen your hand and shoulder muscles. This exercise also increases circulation in the hands and arms and helps improve the flexibility and mobility of wrist joints.

Step-by-Step Instructions

- Sit up tall and comfortable towards the edge of the chair with your spine erect and relaxed, feet flat on the floor at about hip-width apart, and a straight back.

- Rest your hands on your upper thighs just above your knees and take a deep breath in through your nose and slowly exhale.

- Extend both arms straight out in front of you.

- Extend your hands farther from the wrists so that your palms are facing away from you

- Flex your hands from the wrists to turn your palms so that they face your chest

- Repeat.

Elbow Extensions

This exercise helps increase circulation in your arms and shoulders, improve elbow joint mobility and strengthen the muscles in your upper arms and shoulders.

Step-by-Step Instructions

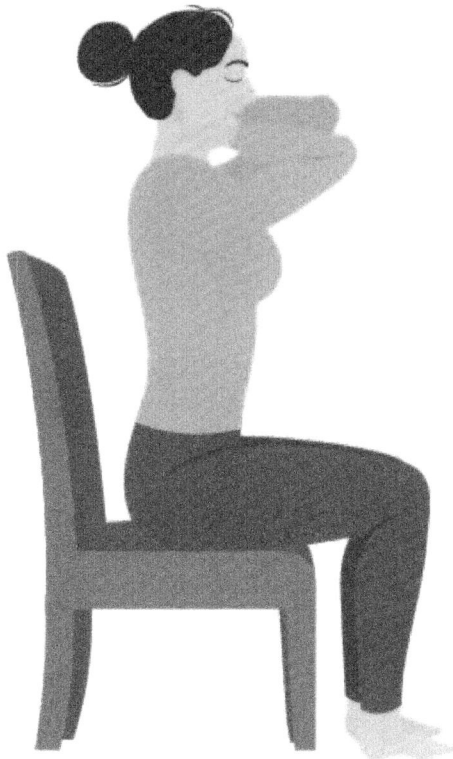

- Sit up tall and comfortable towards the edge of the chair with your spine erect and relaxed, feet flat on the floor at about hip-width apart.

- Rest your hands on your upper thighs just above your knees and take a deep breath in through your nose and slowly exhale.

- Extend your arms to your sides with your palms facing forward.

- Lift them as if you are curling your biceps and bring your fingertips to your shoulders

- Repeat.

Shoulder Shrugs

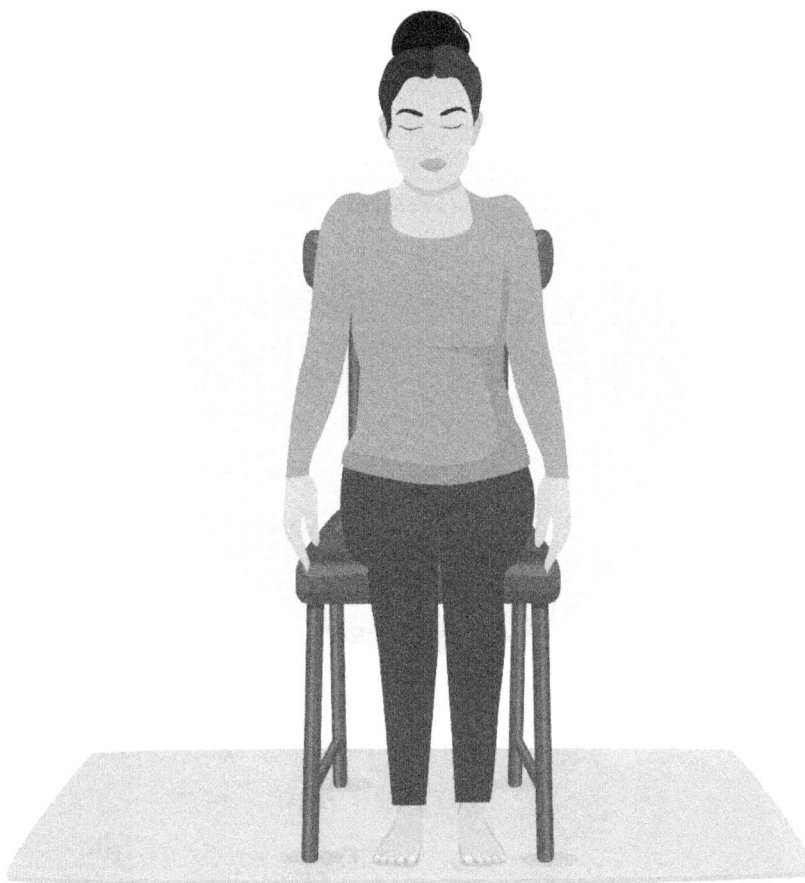

Shoulder shrugs help strengthen your shoulder muscles and promote mobility in your shoulder joints.

Step-by-Step Instructions

- Sit upright in the chair so that your back isn't leaning on the chair
- Keep your feet flat and firmly planted on the floor at a hip distance apart with your palms on your thighs and shoulders relaxed.
- Take a deep breath in through your nose, lifting both shoulders up towards your ears (as if you are freezing cold).
- Hold the tensed position for about three seconds
- Then, release the shoulders fully as you breathe out.
- Repeat.

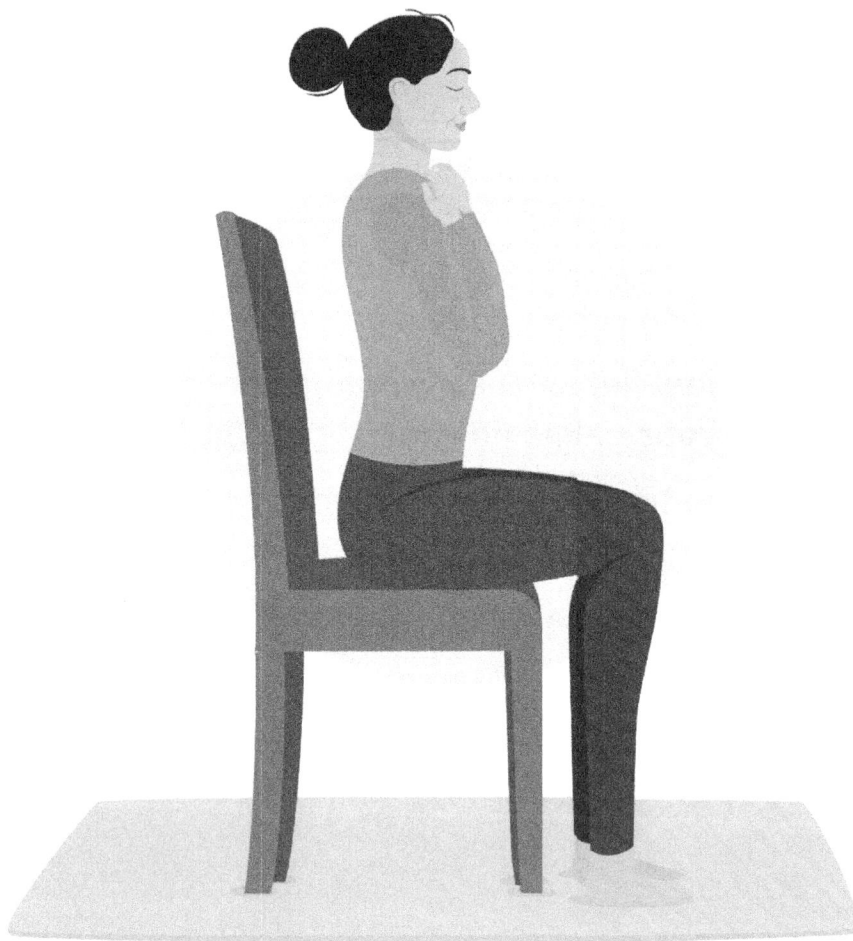

This exercise helps strengthen your upper arm and shoulder muscles. It also increases circulation in your shoulders and improves shoulder joint mobility.

Step-by-Step Instructions

- Sit upright in the chair so that your back isn't leaning on the chair

- Keep your feet flat and firmly planted on the floor at a hip distance apart with your palms on your thighs and shoulders relaxed.

- Bring both hands on your shoulders and hold your shoulder joints with your fingertips.

- Make circles with your elbows starting with moving in a clockwise direction and then anticlockwise.

- Repeat alternating the direction.

Seated Forward Bend

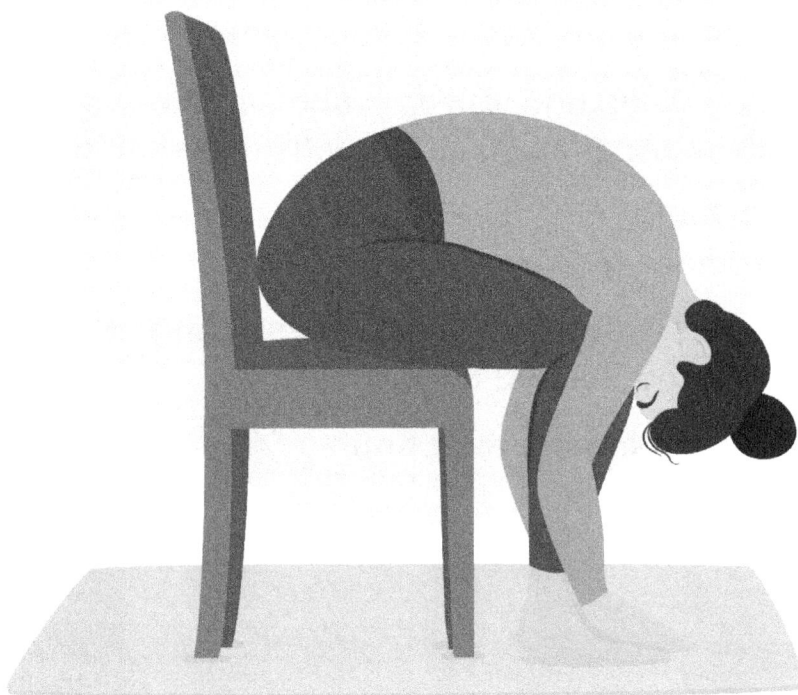

This exercise is helpful in gaining flexibility and mobility in the hips and lower back. It also helps relieve anxiety, stress, and tension.

Step-by-Step Instructions

- Sit up tall in the chair, with your feet planted flat on the floor at a hips distance apart and palms resting on your thighs.

- Take a deep breath in through your nose while lengthening your spine, then exhale as you slowly and gently drop your torso down and let your belly rest on your thighs.

- Lower your hands and touch the floor on your palms.

- Keep your neck relaxed and release your head hanging down

- Hold there for 3-5 deep inhales and exhales

- Then, press your arms gently into the floor and lift your torso slowly to return to a seated position.

- Repeat.

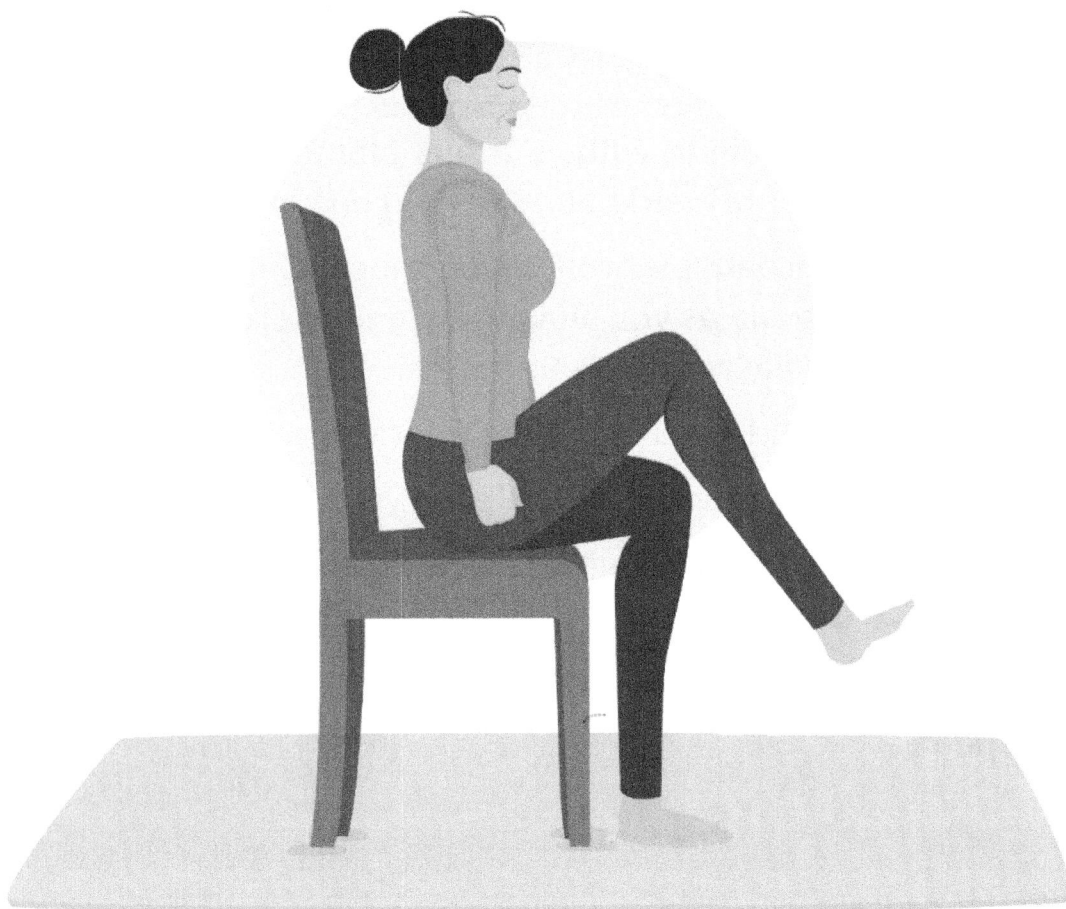

This move helps increase mobility and range of motion in the knees.

Step-by-Step Instructions

- Sit up tall and comfortable in the chair with your spine erect and relaxed, feet flat on the floor at about hip-width apart, belly in, and shoulders back.

- Rest your hands on your laps and take a deep breath in and out through your nose.

- Bring your hands and clasp them under your right knee.

- Sit back upright with a straight spine.

- While holding your hands under your knees, slowly and gently kick the held leg out back and forth. Ensure that you move it through a full range of motion.

- Perform about twenty kicks for each leg.

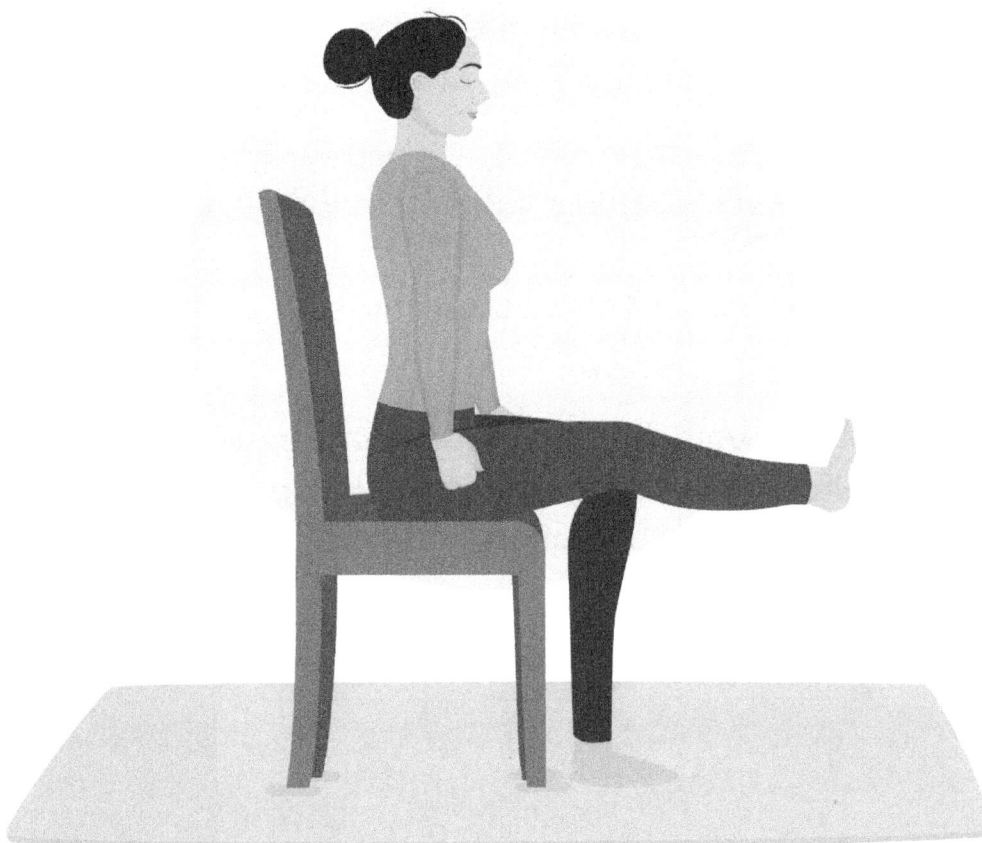

This movement helps strengthen your ankles and improve flexibility and mobility in your ankle joints.

Step-by-Step Instructions

- Sit tall towards the edge of the chair, back straight, and feet flat on the floor at about a hip distance apart.

- Rest your hands on your laps and take a deep breath in and out through your nose.

- Breath in as you extend your right leg straight out in front of you.

- Raise it up and begin rotating its foot clockwise articulating the circles slowly.

- Exaggerate the circles and make them as large as possible.

- Rotate the foot about ten times then switch the direction. Ensure that to keep the lifted leg as straight as possible.

- Rotate the foot in an anticlockwise direction for about ten rotations.

- Switch the legs.

- Repeat alternating between the two legs.

Cooling Pose: Legs on a Chair (Savasana Variation)

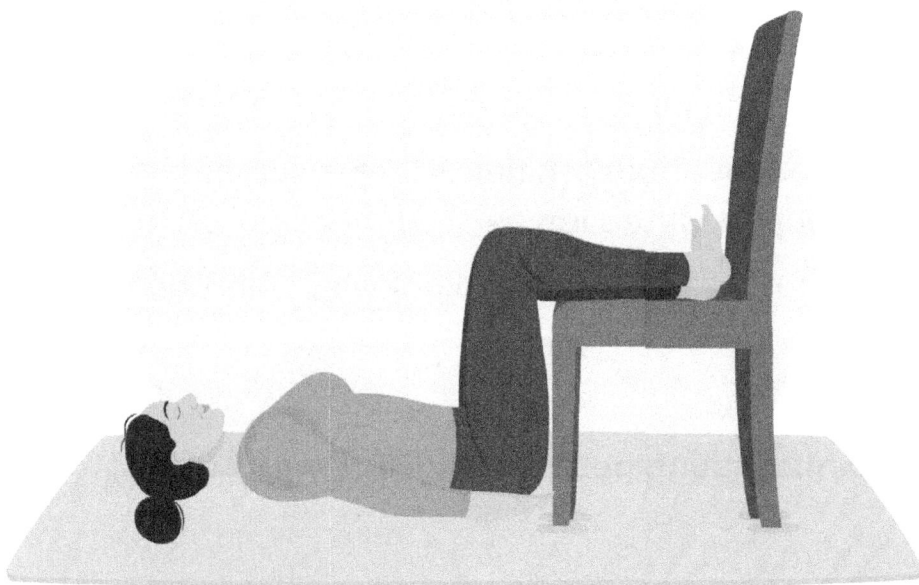

This pose will help your mind calm down, relax your body and unwind.

Step-by-Step Instructions

- Begin by lying down flat on the floor with your hips facing the front of the chair.

- Move your hips close enough to the chair that you can rest your entire lower legs on its seat.

- Place your both legs on the chair ensuring that your calves rest on it comfortably and keep them at a hip distance apart.

- Extend your hands straight out by your sides down on the floor with your palms facing up.

- Close your eyes and take deep breaths

- Pay attention to your breath as you inhale and exhale. Hold here for about 15-25 deep breaths

- To release the pose and come back, open your eyes then slowly and gently remove the legs from the seat.

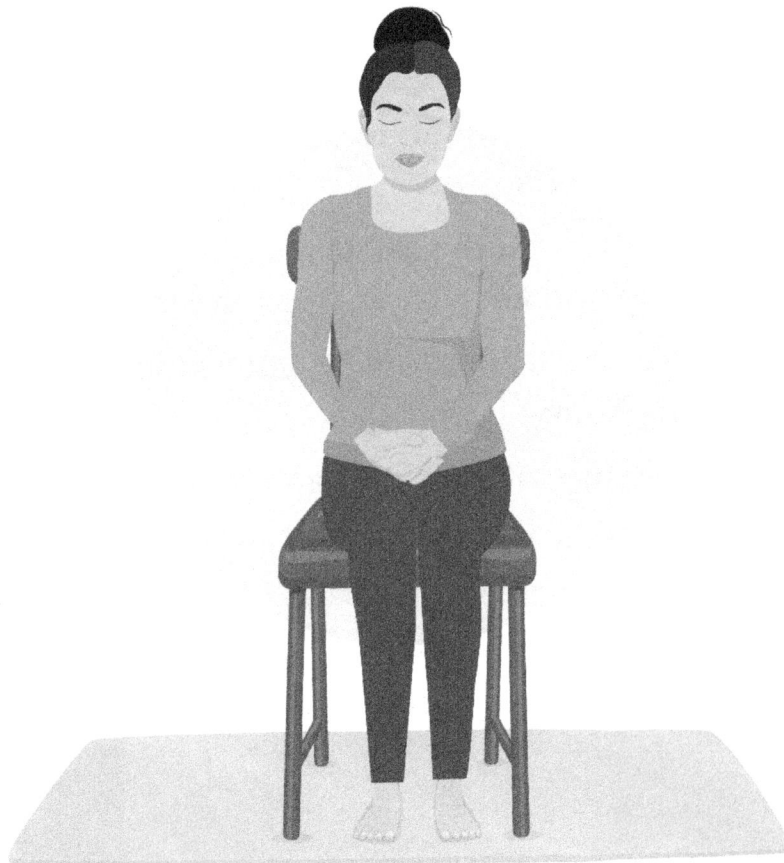

This pose will make you feel good, calm you and give your body time to start integrating the benefits of your yoga practice.

Step-by-Step Instructions

- Sit leaning back comfortably in the chair with your spine against the back of the chair.

- Rest your hands on your laps, relax your hands and close your eyes.

- Keep your entire body relaxed and breathe naturally.

- Pay attention to your relaxed breathing allowing any tension in your body to release.

- Stay in this relaxed position for about three to five minutes.

- Then, slowly open your eyes and wiggle your fingers and toes.

- Get up from the chair in a slow and controlled manner to avoid dizziness.

You are done!

How do you feel?

I hope you feel relaxed and your muscles and joints feel lubricated and ready to move. Try to do this program three to five times every week. We believe that if you are consistent with it and do it for a few weeks you will be ready to move to the intermediate program for osteoarthritis of the hands, hips, and knees discussed in the next chapter. We've referred to it as "intermediate" because the poses here are quite intense and require more stability and balance.

Chapter Seven:
Intermediate Program for Osteoarthritis of the Hands, Knees, and Hips

Here, you will find exercises that are a bit challenging as compared to the ones in the Beginner Program for Osteoarthritis in the previous chapter. Some moves may require you to use some light weights or stand. As usual, before we get started, it is important that we prepare our minds and the breathing system. Let's start with a breathing exercise.

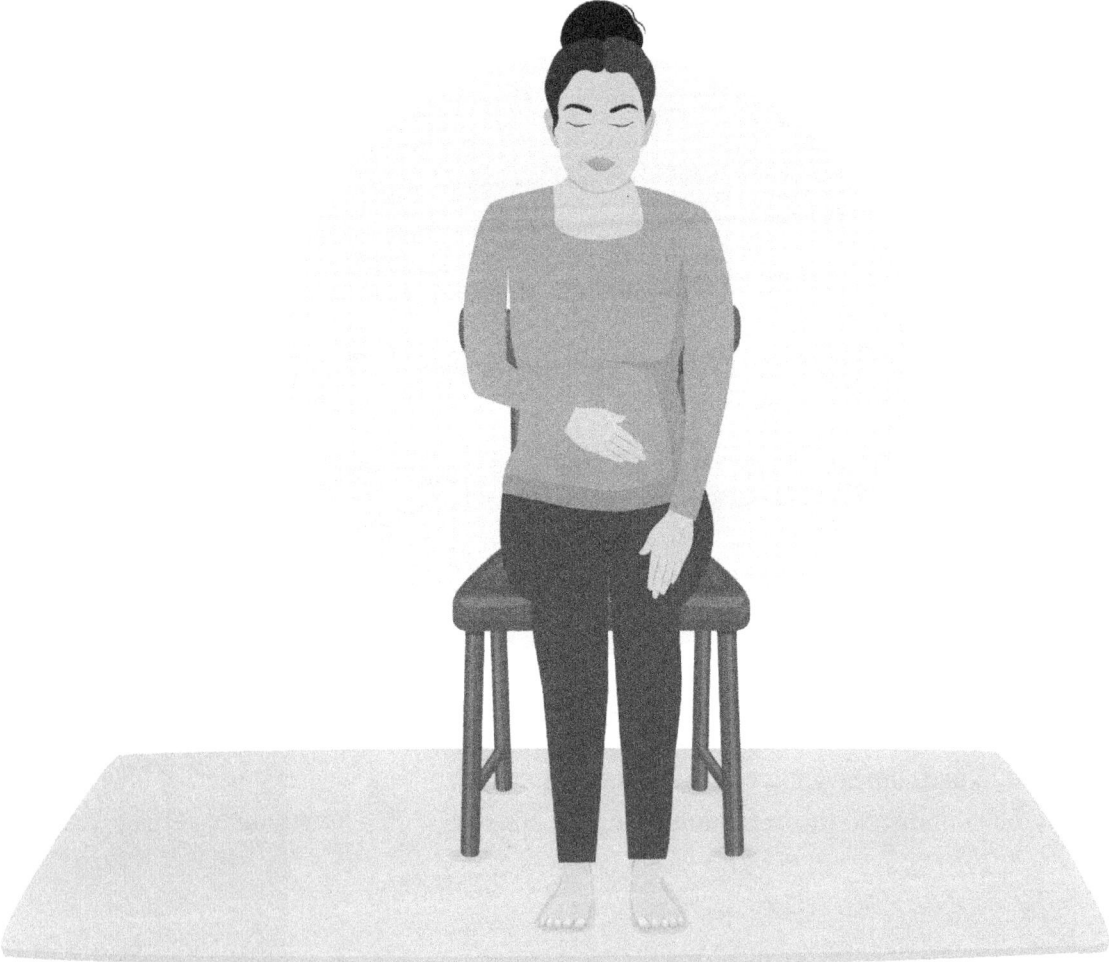

- Sit up tall in the chair leaving some space behind you so that you are not leaning on it.

- Plant your feet flat and firmly on the floor with your hands hanging by your sides

- Keep your left hand relaxed by your side and put your right hand on your belly

- Take a deep full breath in through your nose, then breathe out all the air as you pull your navel and the belly back towards the spine. Next, take a partial breath in and exhale quickly through the nose relaxing the navel and the abdomen. You may pump at a pace of your choice. Just ensure that the breath is continuous but the "breath-ins" are very subtle and small. Perform as many pumps as you can. Start smaller and build your way up.

- On the last pump, stop and take a full breath in and a full breath out.

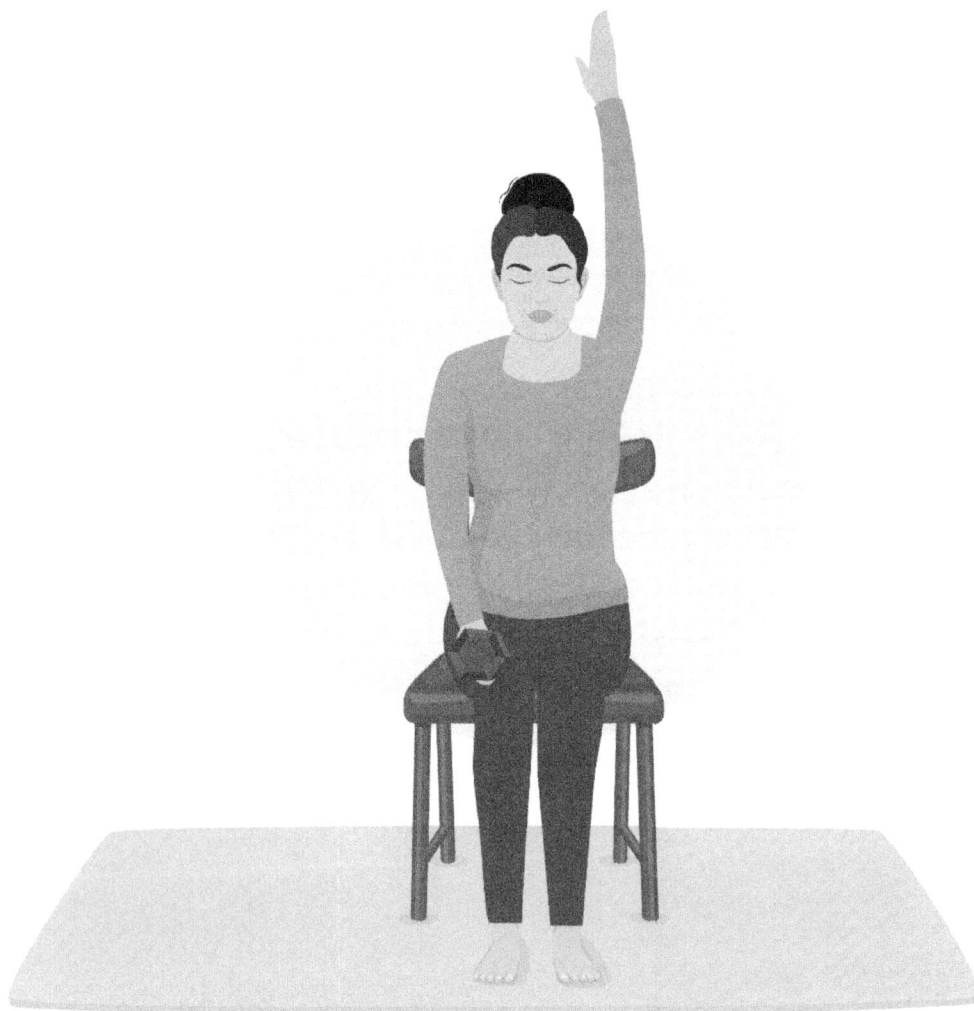

This move helps lubricate your shoulder joint and strengthen your arms.

Step-by-Step Instructions

- Sit tall towards the edge of the chair, with a straight back, and feet flat on the floor at about a hip distance apart.

- Rest your hands on your laps holding two-pound weights and take a deep breath in and out through your nose.

- Breathe in as you lift your right arm above your head. Keep the extended arm as straight as possible and shoulders relaxed.

- Breathe out as you slowly and gently lower the arm back to your thighs.

- Do the same for the left hand.

- Repeat five to ten times on each side.

- On the last rep of each hand, hold the pose and take three full breaths.

Shoulder Rotations

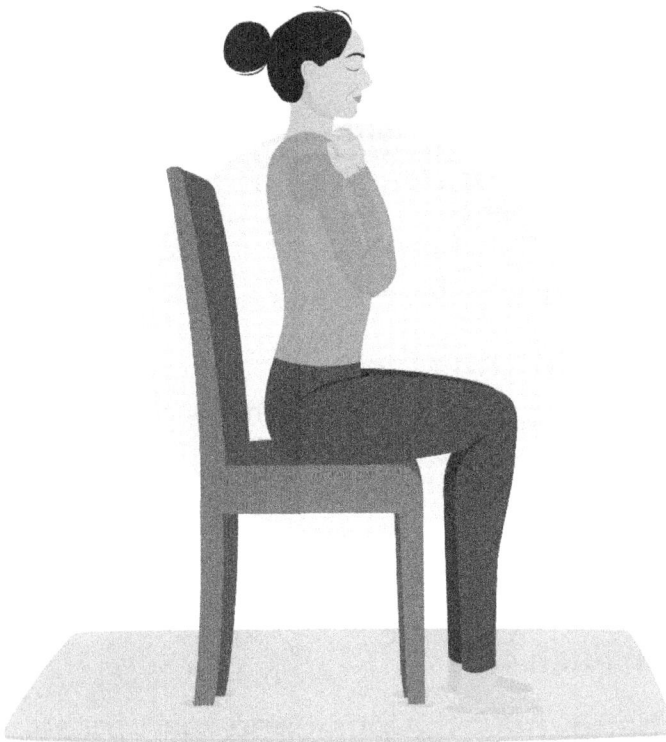

This exercise helps strengthen your upper arm and shoulder muscles. It also improves shoulder joint mobility.

Step-by-Step Instructions

- Sit upright in the chair so that your back isn't leaning on the chair.

- Keep your feet flat and firmly planted on the floor at a hip distance apart with your palms on your thighs and shoulders relaxed.

- Bring both hands on your shoulders and hold your shoulder joints with your fingertips.

- Make circles with your elbows starting with moving in a clockwise direction and then anticlockwise.

- Repeat, alternating the direction.

High Altar Arms

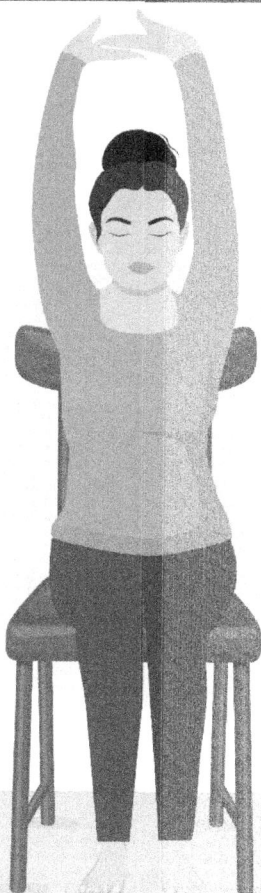

This move works your arms, wrists, shoulders, and the sides of your torso. It helps relieve your arms, shoulders, and wrists from stiffness. It also helps strengthen the muscles in these areas.

Step-by-Step Instructions

- Sit up tall and comfortable towards the edge of the chair with your spine erect and relaxed, feet flat on the floor at about hip-width apart, and a straight back.

- Rest your hands on your upper thighs just above your knees and take a deep breath in through your nose and slowly exhale.

- Extend your arms straight out in front of you, interlace the fingers and keep the palms inverted such that they face away from your torso. Hold here for a few seconds and just feel the stretch.

- Keeping your ribs relaxed, raise your arms up above your head. Ensure that your shoulder tops remain down and stretch from elbow to wrist. Try to imagine that there is something on the altar created above you that you wish to bring into your life.

- Hold here for about 5-10 breaths then release your arms.

- Repeat.

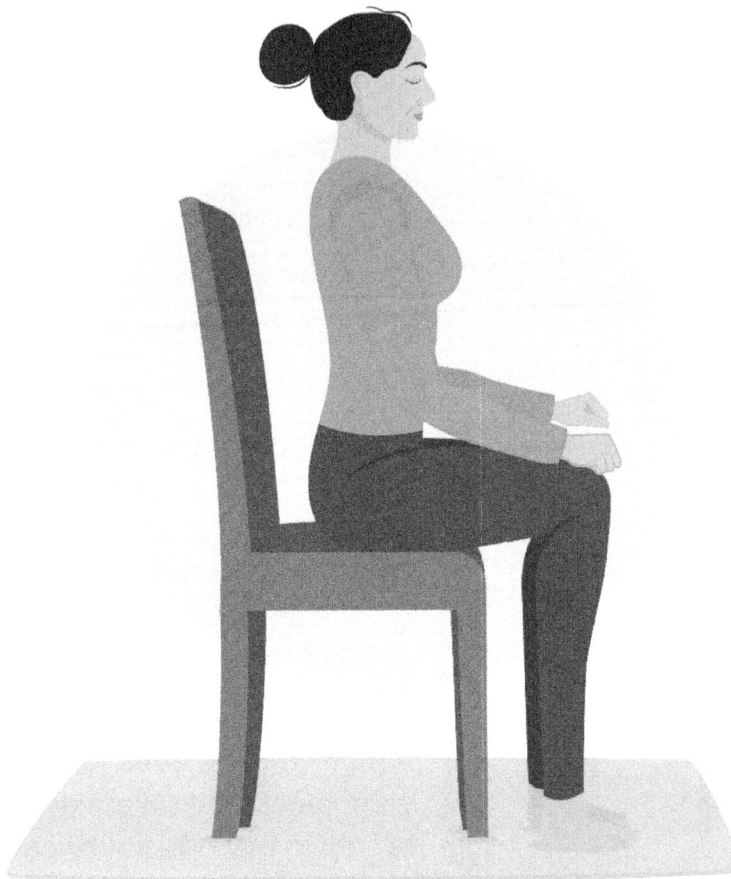

Wrist rotations work out your wrists, hands, and shoulders. They help strengthen your hand and shoulder muscles. This exercise also helps improve the flexibility and mobility of wrist joints.

Step-by-Step Instructions

- Sit up tall and comfortable towards the edge of the chair with your spine erect and relaxed, feet flat on the floor at about hip-width apart, and a straight back.

- Rest your hands on your upper thighs just above your knees and take a deep breath in through your nose and slowly exhale.

- Extend both arms straight out in front of you.

- Rotate your wrists in a clockwise direction, then rotate them in an anticlockwise direction.

- Repeat.

Seated Knee Hugs

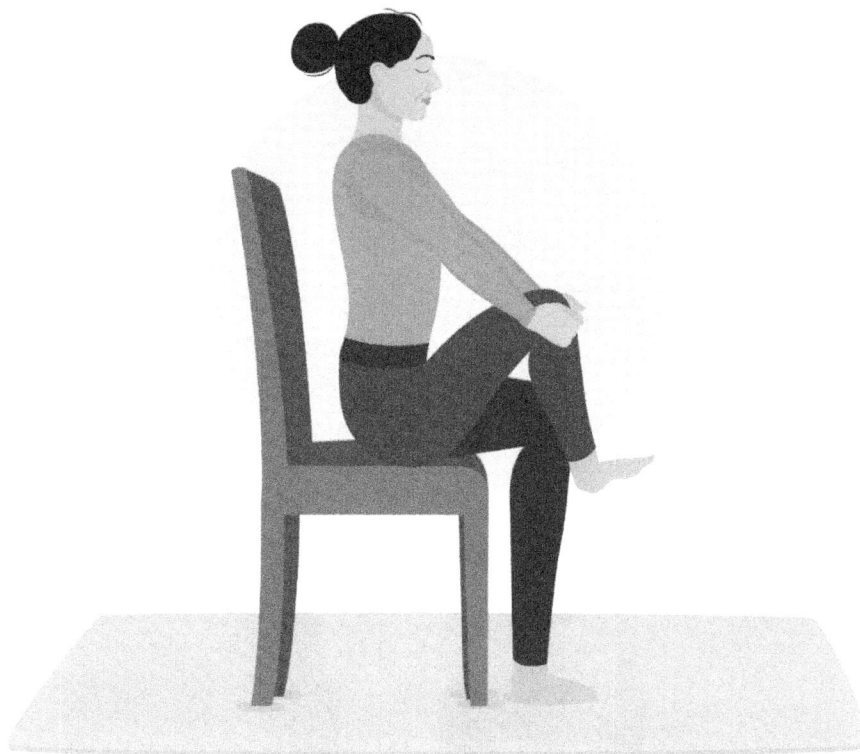

This pose helps strengthen the muscles surrounding your shoulders, legs, and hips. It also improves the mobility and flexibility of the knee and hip joints.

Step-by-Step Instructions

- Sit up tall and comfortable towards the edge of the chair with your spine erect and relaxed, feet planted firmly on the floor at about hip-width apart.

- Rest your hands on your upper thighs just above your knees and take a deep breath in through your nose and slowly exhale.

- Slowly pull your right knee towards your chest.

- Hold there for about 3-5 relaxed breaths.

- Slowly lower the leg down to the floor.

- Repeat for the opposite leg.

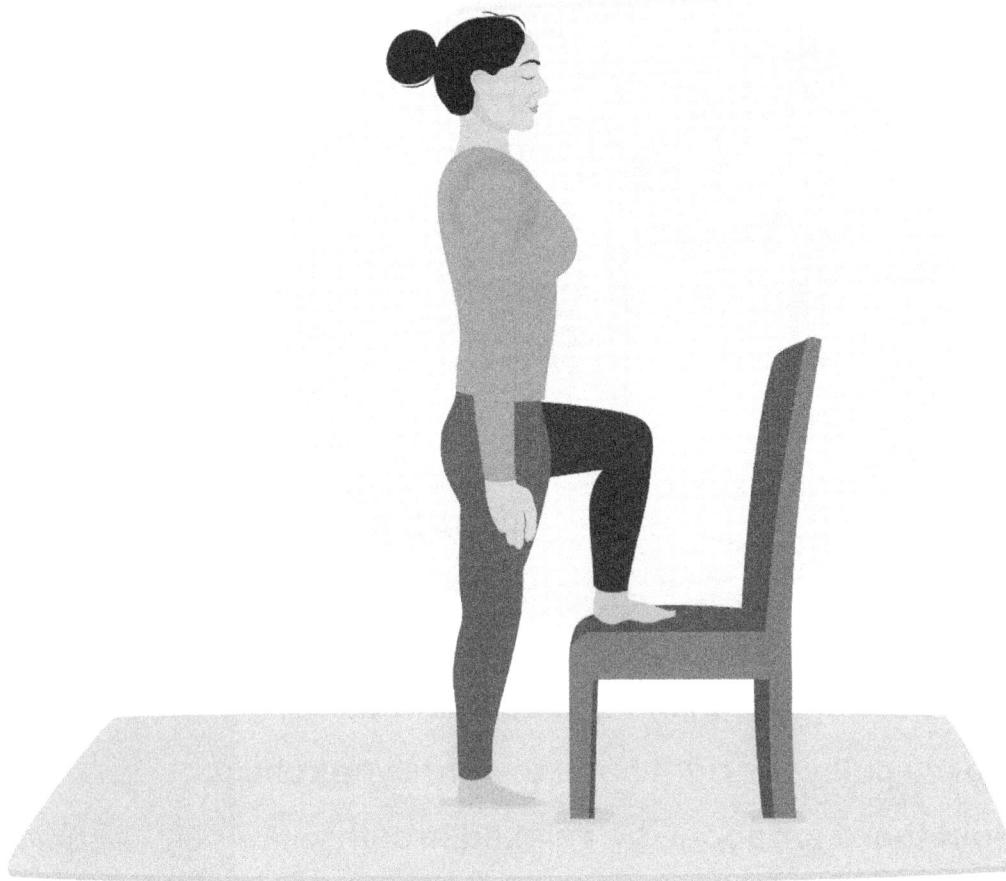

This posture works your hips, knee joints, and legs. It helps improve flexibility and mobility of the hip and knee joints. It also strengthens your leg muscles thus improving your stability and balance.

Step-by-Step Instruction

- Stand up tall in front of the chair with its side facing you. Your feet should be parallel to each other at hip-width apart.

- Take a deep breath in and out then hold the back of the chair with one hand for support. Ensure that you feel stable and relaxed.

- Slowly and mindfully lift the leg that is closest to the chair and put its foot on top of the chair seat. Ensure that your whole foot is on the seat.

- Hold here for a few relaxed breaths. You may try lifting your hand an inch off the chair if you feel your balance is good.

- You may also use a block for placing the foot if the chair is too high and just use the chair for support to hold onto.

- Slowly and gently return the leg to the floor and do the same with the other leg.

- Repeat alternating the legs.

Opposite Leg and Knee Lift (Vyaghrasana Variation)

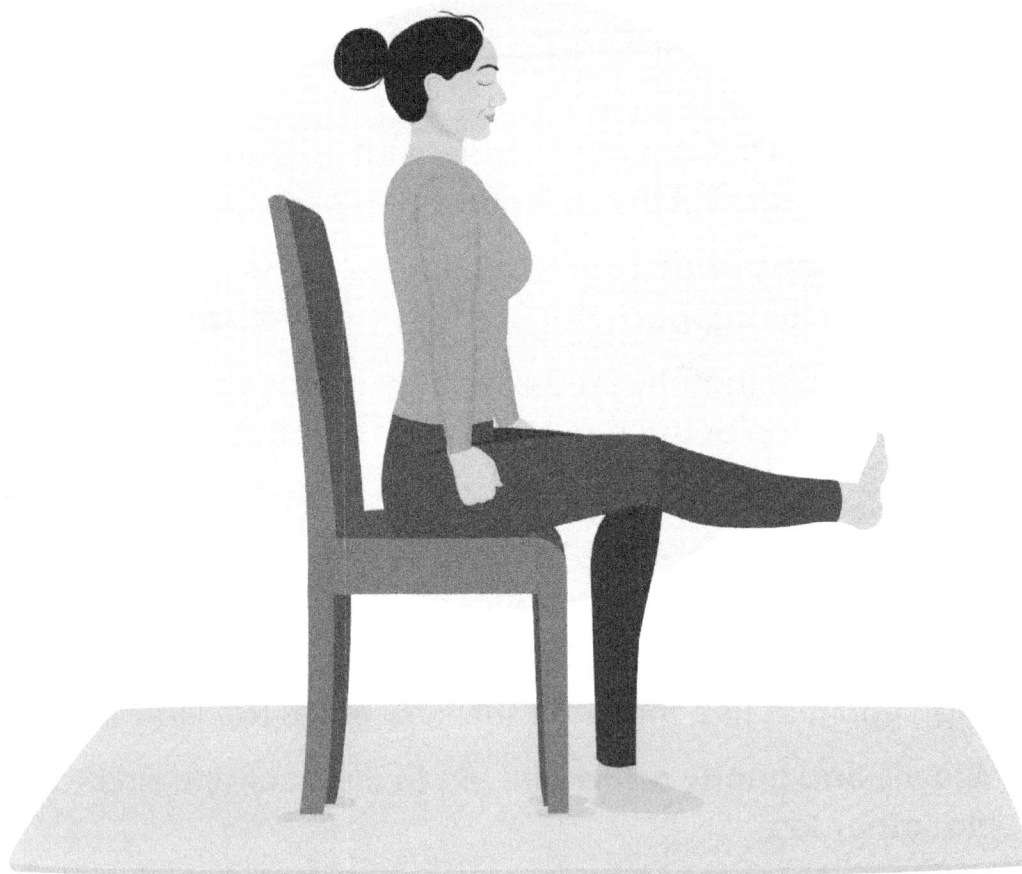

This pose works your hips, knees, abdominals, hamstrings, and quadriceps. It helps strengthen your hips, quadriceps, and abdominals. It also improves mobility in your knee and hip joints.

Step-by-Step Instructions

- Sit tall towards the edge of the chair, with a straight back, and feet flat on the floor at about a hip distance apart.

- Rest your hands on your laps and take a deep breath in and out through your nose.

- Lift your right foot three to five inches off of the ground. Ensure that you keep the foot flexed and parallel to the floor.

- Raise your left arm and extend it straight out in front of you with your palm facing upward.

- Keep your abdominal muscles engaged and hold here for three to five deep breaths.

- Slowly and gently lower your leg and hand back down to release the pose.

- Do the same for the left leg and right hand.

- Repeat five to ten times alternating the legs and hands.

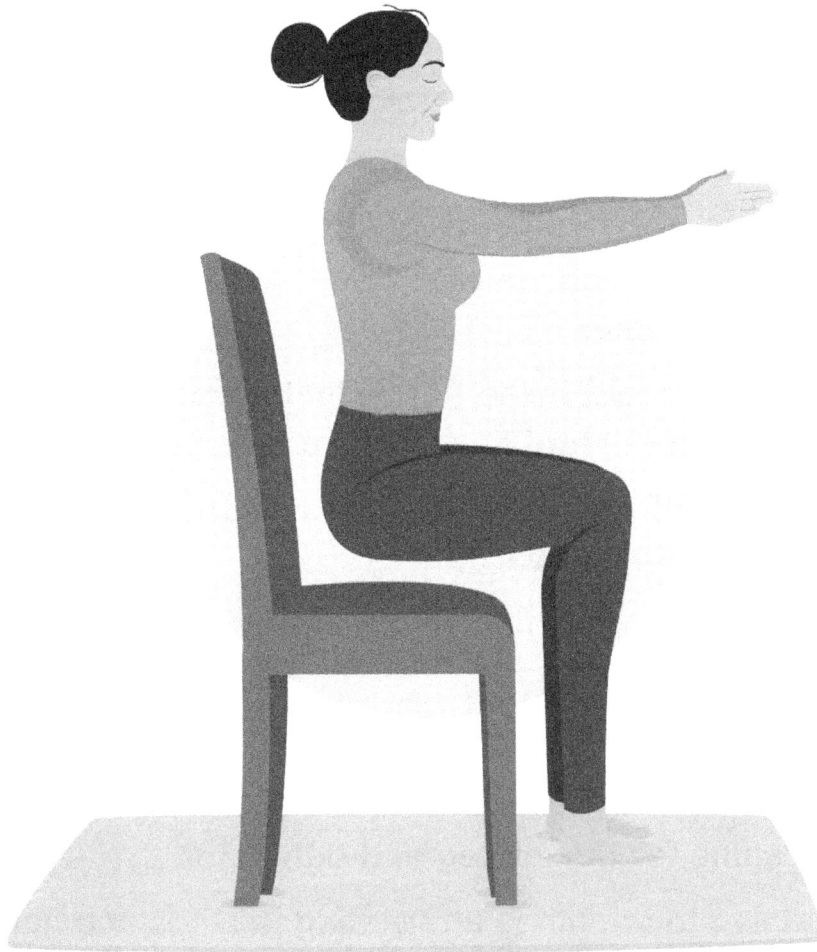

This pose helps strengthen your glutes (the muscles that control sitting down and standing up). It also helps improve your stability and balance.

Step-by-Step Instructions

- Sit tall towards the edge of the chair, with a straight back, and feet flat on the floor at about a hip distance apart.

- Rest your hands on your laps and take a deep breath in and out through your nose.

- Bring your hands down to your sides and bend forward slightly maintaining a straight back and looking straight ahead.

- Now, lift up yourself slowly out of the chair about five inches and extend your arms straight out in front of you. Hold here for two seconds.

- Slowly and gently sit back on the chair in a controlled manner.

- Repeat five to ten times

Seated Twist

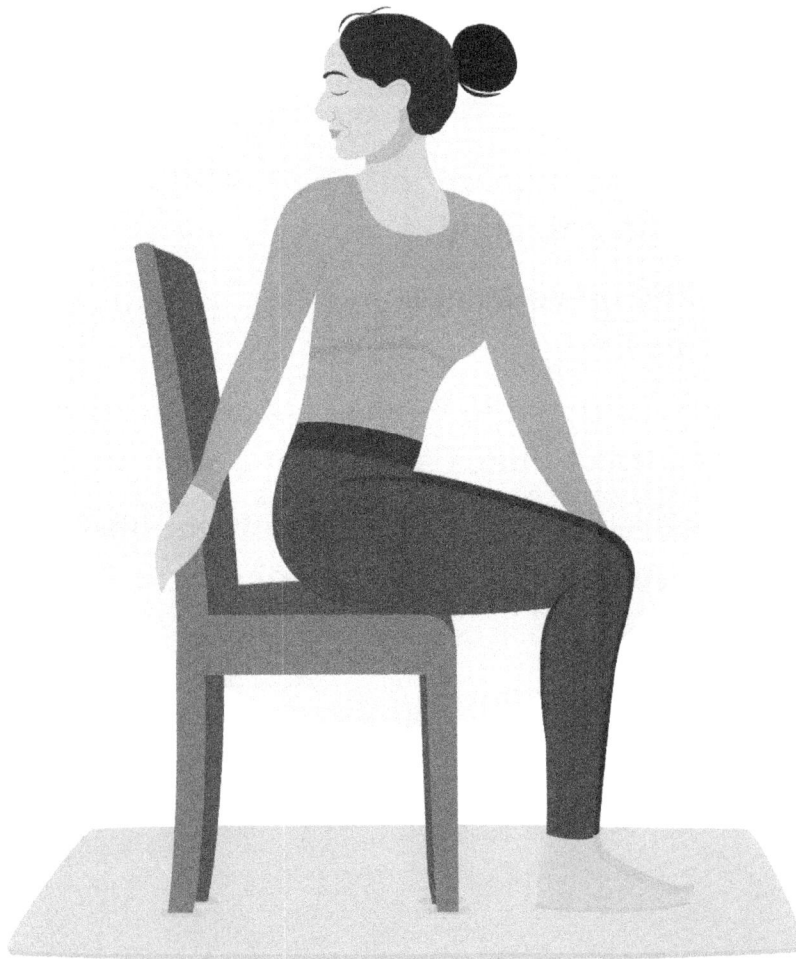

This pose is helpful in gaining flexibility and joint mobility in your hip joints. It also helps relieve stiffness in your arms and hips.

Step-by-Step Instructions

- Sit up tall in the chair leaving some space behind you. Plant your feet flat and firmly on the floor at a hip distance apart with your palms facing down on the upper side of your thighs.

- Take a deep breath in and out then place your left hand on your right thigh and the right hand on the chair seat behind you

- Breathe in as you lengthen your spine, then breathe out and twist your upper body towards the right. Look behind and go as far as you can.

- Hold there for 3-5 deep breaths.

- Unwind from the twist slowly and gently, returning to the center and uncrossing your leg, putting it back on the floor.

- Repeat for the opposite side.

Final Relaxation Pose

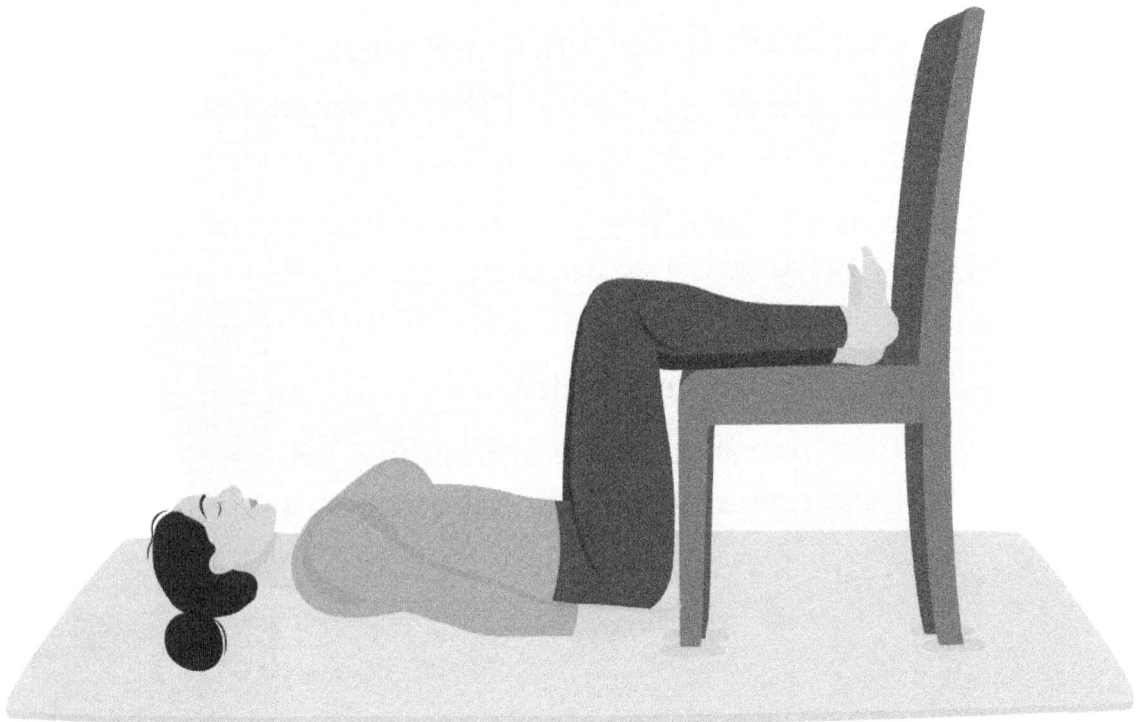

- Begin by lying down flat on the floor with your hips facing the front of the chair.

- Move your hips close enough to the chair that you can rest your entire lower legs on its seat.

- Place your both legs on the chair ensuring that your calves rest on it comfortably and keep them at a hip distance apart.

- Extend your hands straight out by your sides down on the floor with your palms facing up.

- Close your eyes and take deep breaths

- Pay attention to your breath as you inhale and exhale. Hold here for about 15-25 deep breaths

- To release the pose and come back, open your eyes then slowly and gently remove the legs from the seat.

Conclusion

It is never too late to get moving and release stress and stretch every joint and muscle. Don't let the fear of injuries and falls from strength training and high-intensity cardio hold you back from reaping the benefits of staying active in your twilight years. Chair yoga for seniors is a wonderful way to help older citizens prevent old age-related diseases, improve their bodies and keep their minds alert. Now you can enjoy all the benefits of yoga with the program designed in this book.

Never let aching joints overcome you. Pick a routine that best fits your needs and works for you. If you are not sure if the routine will work for you, just try it to see. If you feel it is very easy, move to the most challenging routine. Remember, consistency is key. I encourage you to make your chair yoga workouts a habit and stick with them. Follow your yoga program at least three times every week. The more consistent you remain, the better you will move and feel.

Congratulations! You have come to the end of this book. I hope that these programs have been enjoyable and useful to you, both as a practice in itself and as a starting point to get you excited about creating your own chair yoga routines. You just got started on an amazing journey that will grant you an opportunity for a happier, healthier, and more purposeful life.

Cheers!

JONATHAN PRICE

is an independent publisher, if you enjoy this book, please consider supporting us by leaving a review!

References

Adkins, C. C., Robinson, O. B., & Stewart, B. L. (2011). *Chair Yoga for You: A Practical Guide* (1st ed.). CreateSpace Independent Publishing Platform.

Bondy, D., Rebar, H. K., & Baker, J. (2020). *Yoga Where You Are: Customize Your Practice for Your Body and Your Life* (1st ed.). Shambhala.

Coffin, N. (2013). *Chair Yoga For Seniors: A Gentle Sequence to Get You Started.* UNKOWN.

D'Arrigo, C. (2021). *Chair Yoga: Accessible Sequences to Build Strength, Flexibility, and Inner Calm.* Rockridge Press.

Donovan, S. (2022). *10-Minute Workouts for Seniors 60+: Simple Illustrated Exercises Elderly of Any Level Can Do at Home to Drastically Improve Balance, Strength and Whole-Body Wellness | 4-Week Plan Included.* Independently published.

Egoscue, J. (2022). *5-Minutes Chair Yoga for Seniors: Simple Exercises to Reset The Whole Body.* Independently published.

E-Ryt, C. K. M., Krucoff, C., PhD, C. J., & Md, M. K. W. (2016). *Relax into Yoga for Seniors: A Six-Week Program for Strength, Balance, Flexibility, and Pain Relief* (Illustrated ed.). New Harbinger Publications.

Harvard Health. (2022). *Yoga: Another way to prevent osteoporosis?* https://www.health.harvard.edu/womens-health/yoga-another-way-to-prevent-osteoporosis

Hunter, S. K. (2014). Sex differences in human fatigability: mechanisms and insight to physiological responses. *Acta Physiologica, 210*(4), 768–789. https://doi.org/10.1111/apha.12234

Lehmkuhl, L. (2020). *Chair Yoga for Seniors: Stretches and Poses that You Can Do Sitting Down at Home* (Illustrated ed.). Skyhorse.

Martel, G. F., Roth, S. M., Ivey, F. M., Lemmer, J. T., Tracy, B. L., Hurlbut, D. E., Metter, E. J., Hurley, B. F., & Rogers, M. A. (2006). Age and sex affect human muscle fibre adaptations to heavy-resistance strength training. *Experimental Physiology*, *91*(2), 457–464. https://doi.org/10.1113/expphysiol.2005.032771

Mayer, K. (2022). *Chair Yoga For Seniors & Beginners: Sit N Fit Chair Yoga For Seniors Over 60, Stretches and Poses For Pain Relief, Joint Health, Relaxation, Flexibility*. Independently published.

McBride, A. (2020). *STRETCHING FOR BEGINNERS TO STAY YOUNG: Stretches and Poses that You Can Do Sitting Down at Home to Regain Fitness for women and men over 50*. Independently published.

McGee, K. (2017). *Chair Yoga: Sit, Stretch, and Strengthen Your Way to a Happier, Healthier You* (1st ed.). William Morrow Paperbacks.

Morales, S. (2021). *Chair Yoga for Beginners: The Complete Guide to Easy Yoga Sequences and Poses Suitable for Every Age That You Can Do Sitting at Home in 10 Minutes to Improve Strength, Flexibility, and Calmness*. Independently published.

Obrien, M. (2020). *Chair yoga for seniors: yoga for seniors over 60, Mindful Chair Yoga Poses for home practice - Senior beginners, Chair yoga for beginners*. Independently published.

O'Hagan, F., Sale, D., MacDougall, J., & Garner, S. (1995). Response to Resistance Training in Young Women and Men. *International Journal of Sports Medicine*, *16*(05), 314–321. https://doi.org/10.1055/s-2007-973012

Publications, Golden Lion, & Prayogo, H. (2021). *The New You: The Only Chair Yoga For Seniors Program You'll Ever Need*. Independently published.

Rissanen, J., Walker, S., Pareja-Blanco, F., & Häkkinen, K. (2022). Velocity-based resistance training: do women need greater velocity loss to maximize adaptations? *European Journal of Applied Physiology*, *122*(5), 1269–1280. https://doi.org/10.1007/s00421-022-04925-3

Scott, J. (2022). *Chair Exercises For Seniors: A Comprehensive Guide on Stretches and Poses You Can Do Sitting Down At Home*. Independently published.

Shifroni, E. (2014). *A Chair for Yoga: A complete guide to Iyengar Yoga practice with a chair* (2nd ed.). CreateSpace Independent Publishing Platform.

Singh, D. (2006). Universal Allure of the Hourglass Figure: An Evolutionary Theory of Female Physical Attractiveness. *Clinics in Plastic Surgery*, *33*(3), 359–370. https://doi.org/10.1016/j.cps.2006.05.007

Staron, R. S., Hagerman, F. C., Hikida, R. S., Murray, T. F., Hostler, D. P., Crill, M. T., Ragg, K. E., & Toma, K. (2000). Fiber Type Composition of the Vastus Lateralis Muscle of Young Men and Women. *Journal of Histochemistry & Cytochemistry, 48*(5), 623–629. https://doi.org/10.1177/002215540004800506

Vehrs, P., & Hager, R. (2006). Assessment and Interpretation of Body Composition in Physical Education. *Journal of Physical Education, Recreation & Dance, 77*(7), 46–51. https://doi.org/10.1080/07303084.2006.10597907

Wang, W. L., Chen, K. H., Pan, Y. C., Yang, S. N., & Chan, Y. Y. (2020). The effect of yoga on sleep quality and insomnia in women with sleep problems: a systematic review and meta-analysis. *BMC Psychiatry, 20*(1). https://doi.org/10.1186/s12888-020-02566-4

Wellness-Related Use of Common Complementary Health Approaches Among Adults: United States, 2012. (2012). NCCIH. https://www.nccih.nih.gov/research/wellness-related-use-of-common-complementary-health-approaches-among-adults-united-states-2012

Made in the USA
Monee, IL
29 December 2022